The Science of Herbal Antivirals

Emerging Trends in Natural Viral Defense Mechanisms

Alex Thorn

Table of Contents

INTRODUCTION

In the continuous fight against viral illnesses, researchers and medical professionals are investigating various therapeutic modalities to find effective antiviral medicines. Herbal medicine is a reputable and evolving discipline that offers a diverse range of natural chemicals that may have antiviral effects. "The Science of Herbal Antivirals: Emerging Trends in Natural Viral Defense Mechanisms" bridges traditional herbal practices and state-of-the-art scientific discoveries to investigate this fascinating field thoroughly.

This book is more than just anecdotal evidence or a collection of herbal wisdom, as the title would imply. Instead, it thoroughly analyzes the scientific theories behind herbal antivirals, emphasizing new directions and cutting-edge studies.

A fundamental understanding of viruses and the immune system is at the core of our investigation. We explore the complex molecular pathways viruses utilize to enter host cells, multiply, and avoid being recognized by the immune system. In parallel, we investigate the immune system's dynamic reactions, emphasizing its exceptional capacity to identify and eliminate viral threats. By looking at it this way, we can see how herbal antivirals could affect these mechanisms and strengthen the body's defenses against viral invaders.

The bioactive chemicals in medicinal herbs, which form the basis of herbal antiviral therapy, are central to our topic. We analyze their chemical compositions, clarify their modes of action, and assess their effectiveness using a scientific framework. Discovering powerful antiviral agents that are just waiting to be used for medicinal purposes, we set out on a journey through the various pharmacopeia of nature, starting with well-known herbs like echinacea and elderberry and ending with lesser-known botanicals like Andrographis paniculata and Astragalus membranaceus.

This book covers many subjects as we go through the chapters, from safety concerns and regulatory frameworks to pharmacokinetics and clinical applications. We encounter opportunities as well as obstacles in the process of incorporating herbal medicine into traditional healthcare. In the end, "The Science of Herbal Antivirals" aims to foster a greater understanding of the benefits that may be obtained from combining innovation and tradition, opening the door to a more comprehensive strategy for preventing and treating viral diseases.

CHAPTER I

Understanding Viruses and Immunity

Virology Essentials

The study of viruses, which are the tiniest infectious agents known to science, is known as virology. A thorough investigation of viral structure, reproduction, classification, and the dynamic interactions that occur between viruses and their hosts is at the core of virology. It is essential for the general public, researchers, and medical professionals to understand the fundamentals of virology, particularly in light of new infectious illnesses and global pandemics.

Even though they are simpler and smaller than other microbes, viruses are remarkably adept at infecting and controlling host cells for their own benefit. Viruses are primarily made up of a nucleic acid genome, which can be either DNA or RNA, covered in a protein known as a capsid. During the budding process, several viruses additionally enclose themselves in a lipid membrane that originates from the host cell. This fundamental structure is crucial to the replication and spread of viruses and varies significantly throughout viral families.

Viruses typically go through multiple distinct stages in their replication cycle, all of which are meticulously arranged to aid in the creation of new viral particles. Viral attachment, the initial stage, allows the virus to enter the host cell through specific interactions between viral surface proteins and also host cell receptors. The process involves multiple stages, namely penetration, replication, assembly, and release when the viral DNA is released into the host cell. During replication, the genetic material of the virus is copied, and new components are synthesized.

Lastly, when the mature virions are released from the host cell, they infect nearby cells or new hosts.

Viral variety is one of the most exciting areas in virology. Because viruses have such a diverse range of sizes, shapes, and genetic makeup, they are categorized into several families, genera, and species according to the traits they have in common. Certain viruses, for instance, have an easy-to-understand icosahedral or helical capsid structure, whilst other viruses have more intricate structures, including filamentous or enclosed forms.

Moreover, viruses exhibit remarkable adaptability and evolutionary power due to their capacity to infect a diverse array of hosts, such as bacteria, fungi, plants, animals, and even other viruses.

A virus's nucleic acid type (DNA or RNA), strandedness (double- or single-stranded), genome size, and replication mechanism are among the factors that determine its classification. Virus nomenclature and classification are overseen by the International Committee on Taxonomy of Viruses, also known as ICTV, to ensure accuracy and consistency in viral taxonomy.

In addition to offering a framework for comprehending the evolutionary links between various viruses, this hierarchical classification approach facilitates the creation of potent antiviral treatments.

Viruses have a significant role in human health and disease, in addition to being infectious agents. Globally, viral infections are a significant cause of mortality and morbidity, ranging from minor colds to severe diseases like AIDS, Ebola, and COVID-19. The creation of treatment approaches, diagnostic procedures, and preventive measures all depend on an understanding of the underlying virology of these illnesses.

Additionally, there are connections between virology and immunology, epidemiology, and molecular biology. For example, the host immune response to viral infections is critical in determining the course of the illness and the emergence of immunity. To monitor the transmission of viral illnesses and carry out public health interventions to contain outbreaks, epidemiologists rely on virological data. Molecular biologists use virological tools to investigate the molecular aspects of viral gene expression, replication mechanisms, and viral-host interactions.

Our capacity to treat viral diseases advances along with our comprehension of virology. The discipline has undergone a revolution thanks to technological advancements like genome editing, structural biology, and next-generation sequencing, which have allowed researchers to study viral biology in unprecedented detail and accuracy. Multinational cooperation and data-sharing programs have also made it easier to respond quickly to new viral threats. This is demonstrated by the multinational efforts made to create vaccines against SARS-CoV-2, the virus that caused the COVID-19 pandemic.

In summary, virology essentials cover a wide range of subjects, including the fundamental structure and replication of viruses as well as their diversity, classification, and effects on human health. Researchers and medical practitioners can learn a great deal about the mechanics of viral pathogenesis and create novel treatments and preventative measures for viral diseases by exploring the complexities of viral biology. Virology is at the forefront of scientific study and guides our efforts to prevent infectious diseases and protect public health even when new viral threats emerge.

The Dynamic Immune Response

The immune system is an excellent biological defensive system that keeps the body safe from a variety of pathogens, such as parasites, viruses, bacteria, and fungi. Fundamentally, the immune response is a dynamic and intricately planned process that combines the coordinated actions of several chemicals, tissues, and cells. The immune response is defined by its capacity to change and adapt in response to evolving threats, from the first recognition of invasive pathogens to the production of specialized immune cells and the final resolution of infection.

Innate immunity and also adaptive immunity are the two primary branches into which the immune response can be roughly divided. The body's first line of defense against infection is called innate immunity, which is based on a collection of defense systems that are quickly activated when pathogens are encountered. The skin and mucous membranes, as well as cellular elements, including neutrophils and dendritic cells, including macrophages, are essential parts of the innate immune system. Pathogen-associated molecular patterns (PAMPs) are conserved molecular patterns found on the surface of pathogens that are recognized by the aforementioned cells' pattern recognition receptors (PRRs).

Innate immunity cells recognize PAMPs and set off a series of immune responses that include pro-inflammatory cytokine release, immune cell recruitment to the infection site, and antimicrobial mechanism activation to eradicate invasive pathogens.

On the other hand, the immune system's more complex and specialized component, known as adaptive immunity, offers persistent defense against particular infections. T cells and B cells, among other lymphocytes, are involved in adaptive immunity. They expand and select clonally to produce antigen-specific effector cells that can identify and destroy invasive infections. Immunological memory is a critical idea in adaptive immunity, whereby the immune system remembers previous infections it has encountered in order to mount a more vigorous and faster defense when it is reexposed. Vaccination, the cornerstone of contemporary medicine that uses the immune system to prevent infectious diseases, is based on this memory.

The immune response's capacity to change and adapt in response to evolving threats is a clear indication of its dynamic character. Numerous processes, including immunological evasion, immune modulation, and antigenic diversity, contribute to this flexibility. The term "antigenic variation" describes a pathogen's capacity to alter its surface antigens in order to avoid being recognized by the immune system. This makes it possible for viruses to evade the immune system's detection and elimination, which can result in persistent or recurring infections. Conversely, immune evasion describes a pathogen's capacity to thwart or inhibit the host immune response, which enables the infection to start and continue. Immune evasion can be accomplished by pathogens through a variety of strategies, such as the release of immunomodulatory substances, the suppression of immune cell activity, or the interference with signaling cascades that lead to immune activation.

Apart from safeguarding against infectious illnesses, the immune response is essential for preserving tissue equilibrium and averting autoimmunity. Chronic inflammation and tissue damage result from the immune system attacking the body's own tissues by mistake, a condition known as autoimmune disease. The immune system uses a number of immune tolerance mechanisms, such as peripheral tolerance in peripheral tissues, central tolerance in the thymus and bone marrow, and the ability of regulatory T cells (Tregs) to dampen overactive immune responses to prevent autoimmunity. These defense mechanisms let the immune system distinguish between self and non-self and mount an effective fight against invasive intruders, all the while limiting harmful immune reactions against the body's own tissues.

Numerous environmental elements can affect the immune response, including host genetics, microbial diversity, and lifestyle elements like exercise and nutrition. For instance, it has been demonstrated that the gut microbiota's makeup affects how the immune system develops and functions, influencing immunological responses and a person's vulnerability to inflammatory and infectious diseases. In a similar vein, the genetic makeup of the host can affect both the severity of immune-mediated diseases and the susceptibility to infectious diseases. Studies indicate that a good diet and regular exercise can improve immune function and lower the risk of viral and inflammatory disorders. Lifestyle factors like food and exercise can also have a substantial impact on immune function.

To sum up, the immune response is a biological defensive mechanism that is dynamic and highly flexible. It is essential for defending the body against viral illnesses, preserving tissue homeostasis, and averting autoimmunity. The immune response is defined by its capacity to change and adapt in response to evolving threats, from the first recognition of invasive pathogens to the production of specialized immune cells and the final resolution of infection. By deciphering the complexities of immune response and immune response-influencing factors, scientists can learn more about the mechanisms behind immunological-mediated diseases and create innovative approaches to diagnosis, therapy, and prevention. In the end, developing a greater comprehension of the dynamic immune response is essential to opening up fresh possibilities for therapeutic intervention and enhancing human health and well-being.

Interplay between Viruses and Immune System

A complicated and dynamic process that changes the course of viral infections and affects the result of host-pathogen interactions is the interaction between viruses and the immune system. Viruses are intracellular parasites that depend on their host cells for both survival and reproduction. To detect and eradicate viral infections, on the other hand, the immune system has developed highly developed mechanisms that restrict the harmful effects of viruses and stop them from spreading. Comprehending the dynamic between viruses and the immune system is imperative in order to clarify the processes involved in viral pathogenesis, create efficacious vaccines and antiviral treatments, and ultimately manage viral infections.

The immunological response to viral infections is coordinated by the combined action of the innate and also adaptive immune systems. The primary defense mechanism against viral infections is the innate immune response, which is quick yet nonspecific. Pattern recognition receptors (PRRs) on innate immune cells, such as macrophages, dendritic cells, and also natural killer (NK) cells, identify conserved molecular patterns on the surface of viruses, or pathogen-associated molecular patterns (PAMPs), as indicators of the presence of viral pathogens. Innate immune cells recognize PAMPs and set off a series of immunological responses that include recruiting more immune cells to the infection site, releasing pro-inflammatory cytokines, and activating antimicrobial mechanisms to eradicate invasive viruses.

Simultaneously, the adaptive immune response responds to viral infections in a more targeted and focused manner. T cells and B cells, among other lymphocytes, mediate this response by going through a clonal selection and expansion process that produces effector cells specific to an antigen that can identify and eradicate the invasive viruses. The idea of immunological memory, which states that the immune system remembers previous viral contacts and uses that information to mount a more robust and faster defense when exposed to the same virus again, is essential to adaptive immunity. Vaccination, the cornerstone of contemporary medicine that uses the immune system's ability to create long-lasting protective immunity in order to prevent viral infections, is based on this memory.

A set of dynamic interactions characterizes the interplay between viruses and the immune system, influencing the course of viral infections. Viruses have developed a number of evasive or manipulative tactics to get past the host immune system and continue to infect. To avoid being discovered and eliminated by the immune system, certain viruses, for instance, encode proteins that block the host's antiviral immunological reactions, such as interferon signaling pathways. In order to elude immune monitoring or to facilitate viral multiplication and dissemination, other viruses may alter the functions of host cells. Furthermore, viruses can change their surface proteins through a process known as antigenic variation, which allows them to evade the host's immune system and cause repeated or chronic infections.

On the other hand, the immune system has developed defense mechanisms to identify and get rid of viral infections, which stops viruses from spreading and stops illness from occurring. For instance, by identifying and eliminating cells that have viral antigens on their surface, cytotoxic T lymphocytes (CTLs) contribute significantly to the removal of virus-infected cells. Similar to this, B cell-produced neutralizing antibodies have the ability to attach to viral particles and stop them from infecting host cells, therefore preventing viral spread and accelerating viral clearance. Furthermore, the immune system has the capacity to produce durable immune memory against particular viruses, shielding populations from future infections and promoting herd immunity.

Age, underlying medical conditions, genetics, and other host characteristics all have an impact on how viruses interact with the immune system. The degree of immune-mediated illnesses and the susceptibility to viral infections can both be influenced by host genetic variables. For instance, some genetic variations in the genes that code for immune-related proteins may make a host more vulnerable to viral infections or change how the host's immune system reacts to viral infections. Furthermore, immunosenescence and other age-related immune system modifications might impair the host's capacity to develop a potent defense against viral infections, making older persons more vulnerable to severe illness. Additionally, the immune system's ability to fight off viral infections might be weakened by underlying medical disorders, including immunodeficiency or persistent inflammation, which raises the possibility of consequences.

In summary, the dynamic and complex process of viruses interacting with the immune system determines how viral infections progress and how host-pathogen interactions turn out. Viruses have developed a number of evasive or manipulative tactics to get past the host immune system and continue to infect. To stop the spread of viruses and also lessen their harmful consequences, the immune system has developed complex ways to identify and eradicate viral infections. Comprehending the dynamic between viruses and the immune system is imperative in order to clarify the processes involved in viral pathogenesis, create efficacious vaccines and antiviral treatments, and ultimately manage viral infections.

CHAPTER II

Unveiling Natural Viral Defense Mechanisms

Ancient Wisdom: Herbal Remedies through the Ages

Since ancient times, herbal treatments have been an essential component of human civilization, forming the basis of traditional medical systems in many countries and regions. Herbal medicine has long been used to promote health and well-being, from the ancient civilizations of Mesopotamia, Egypt, and China to the traditional healing methods used by Native American tribes and African societies. Evidence of herbal concoctions from thousands of years ago has been discovered in archeological sites, demonstrating the long history of using therapeutic herbs. Herbal treatments have been used for millennia, handed down through the generations, documented in written books, oral traditions, and empirical knowledge, and customized to suit regional climates and customs. The legacy of ancient wisdom continues to this day in modern herbal medicine, as researchers and practitioners work to uncover the medicinal properties of plants and combine traditional knowledge with cutting-edge science and clinical application.

Herbal treatments played a significant role in the prevention and also the treatment of a wide range of maladies in ancient cultures, from minor ones like headaches and indigestion to more serious ones like infections and chronic disorders. Around 3000 BCE, the Sumerians and Babylonians in Mesopotamia used clay tablets to record the use of medical plants. These tablets contained hundreds of herbal cures for various health issues. Similarly, a wide pharmacopeia of herbal treatments made from plants like frankincense, garlic, and aloe vera were used in ancient Egyptian medicine, as recorded in the Ebers Papyrus and other medical literature. Herbal medicine originated in China, supposedly under the guidance of the legendary Emperor Shen Nong, who is credited with tasting hundreds of different herbs to determine their therapeutic qualities. Traditional Chinese medicine (TCM) is based on ancient Chinese pharmacopoeia, which was collected in books like the Shen Nong Ben Cao Jing. It includes comprehensive descriptions of hundreds of medicinal plants and their therapeutic applications.

Native American societies such as the Inca, Aztec, and Maya civilizations in the Americas created complex herbal medicine systems based on their understanding of local flora and natural resources. For example, the Aztecs cultivated medicinal plants like maize, amaranth, and chia for their therapeutic virtues. At the same time, the Mayans used plants like cacao, vanilla, and chaya for both medicinal and ceremonial uses. Analogously, the Inca society of the Andes Mountains depended on plants such as coca, quinoa, and maca for their nutritional and therapeutic properties, with herbal cures being an essential part of their medical framework. African traditional healers have historically used medicinal plants such as hoodia, rooibos, and African potatoes to treat a variety of illnesses. They do this by using information that has been passed down orally for ages through cultural rituals and customs.

Ancient civilizations made extensive use of herbal treatments, which is a testament to both the wisdom of traditional medical methods and the close bond that exists between humans and also the natural world. Through empirical observation, intuition, and trial-and-error, ancient healers studied the effects of plants on health and well-being, progressively learning about the therapeutic qualities of many plants and their uses in medicine. This information was eventually incorporated into traditional medical systems, which are still in use and revered today. Examples of these systems include traditional African medicine, Unani medicine in the Middle East, and also Ayurveda in India.

The holistic approach to health and also healing that ancient herbal medicine takes, acknowledging the interdependence of the mind, body, and spirit, is one of its defining characteristics. Health, according to ancient healers, was a condition of balance and harmony both inside the individual and with the natural environment rather than only the absence of disease. Herbal medicines were utilized to address the underlying causes of illness and promote well-being on a physical, emotional, as well as spiritual level, in addition to treating specific symptoms. Traditional medical systems like Ayurveda and TCM, which place a strong emphasis on diet, lifestyle, and mental health in preserving health and preventing disease, are prime examples of this holistic viewpoint.

Herbal treatments have persisted as a valuable and traditional method of healthcare despite the development of pharmaceutical medications and modern medicine. Herbal therapy has seen a rise in popularity in recent years as more individuals look for complementary and alternative remedies to traditional medical practices. Numerous traditional herbal medicines have been confirmed by scientific study, which confirms their safety and efficacy for a range of health concerns. For instance, research has demonstrated the anti-inflammatory and immune-boosting qualities of herbs like ginger, turmeric, and echinacea, as well as the mood- and cognitive-improving effects of plants like ginkgo biloba and St. John's wort. In addition, the increased desire from consumers for natural, plant-based therapies that they believe to be safe and effective has led to a surge in the popularity of herbal supplements and natural health products in recent years.

In conclusion, there is much that old knowledge may teach us about the therapeutic value of plants and the long history of herbal therapy. Herbal treatments have been utilized for thousands of years to promote health, prevent disease, and restore balance to the body and mind in many cultures and civilizations. When scientists and practitioners investigate the curative potential of medicinal plants and combine traditional wisdom with cutting-edge research and clinical practice, the knowledge and insights of ancient healers continue to influence and inform modern herbal medicine. It is evident that the wisdom of the past will continue to direct us toward health and healing as we look to the future. They will act as a continual reminder of the interdependent nature of humans and the natural world, as well as the need to preserve ancient healing practices for upcoming generations.

The Rise of Modern Herbal Medicine

Herbal therapy has seen a rise in popularity recently as more individuals look for supplementary and alternative therapies to traditional medical practices. The importance of conventional healing methods and the therapeutic potential of medicinal plants are being recognized by both individuals and healthcare professionals, marking a dramatic shift in healthcare paradigms. The emergence of contemporary herbal medicine is a reflection of people's desire for more natural, holistic approaches to health and also well-being, as well as their growing awareness of the drawbacks and adverse effects of pharmaceutical medications.

The growing amount of scientific evidence demonstrating the safety and effectiveness of herbal medicines is one of the factors propelling the growth of contemporary herbal therapy. Studies examining the pharmacological characteristics, mechanisms of action, and possible therapeutic uses of medicinal plants have proliferated in the last few decades. Numerous medicinal plants, including polyphenols, flavonoids, alkaloids, and terpenes, have been shown to contain bioactive chemicals. These compounds have a variety of biological actions, including anti-inflammatory, antibacterial, anticancer, and antioxidant qualities. Additionally, studies on clinical trials have shown that some herbal treatments, like garlic for cardiovascular health, St. John's wort for depression, and ginger for nausea and vomiting, are helpful in treating particular medical disorders. As a result, herbal supplements, plant extracts, and herbal medicines are becoming more widely accessible and well- liked by both consumers and healthcare professionals, leading to an increased integration of herbal medicine into conventional healthcare systems.

The increasing popularity of holistic health and wellness is another element driving the growth of modern herbal medicine. Many people are turning to natural therapies and lifestyle interventions to improve their general well-being and prevent chronic diseases in today's fast-paced, stressful society. Herbal medicine offers a complete approach to health that considers not only the impact that food, lifestyle choices, and environmental factors play in maintaining and improving health but also the interaction between the mind, body, and spirit. Herbal treatments are frequently utilized to promote long-term health and vitality by addressing the underlying imbalances and causes of illness in addition to symptom relief. Herbal medicine also highlights the significance of customized treatment plans, acknowledging that every individual is different and may react to herbal medicines in different ways depending on their genetic makeup, constitution, and state of health. Many individuals who are looking for alternatives to conventional medicine's one-size-fits-all approach find resonance in this tailored approach to healthcare.

The increased demand from consumers for natural, plant-based therapies that are regarded as mild, safe, and effective is another factor contributing to the emergence of contemporary herbal medicine. Many people are turning to herbal medicine as a more sustainable and ecologically friendly alternative to traditional pharmaceuticals in an era where ecological balance and environmental sustainability are becoming more and more critical. Herbal treatments are made from natural plant sources and may be collected, grown, and processed sustainably with little negative impact on the environment. This is in contrast to synthetic pharmaceuticals, which are frequently made from petrochemicals and require substantial processing and manufacture. Herbal medicine also provides a more ecological and holistic approach to healing, one that honors the interdependence of all living things and the natural world, as well as the fragile equilibrium of ecosystems and biodiversity.

In addition to its therapeutic benefits, modern herbal medicine has become increasingly recognized for its ability to inspire people to take ownership of their own well-being and health. Herbal medicine promotes self-reliance and self-care, as well as a closer bond with nature and the natural world, by arming people with the information and tools necessary to cultivate, harvest, and make their own herbal treatments. Learning about medicinal plants and their traditional applications, growing their own herbal gardens, and being involved in community herbalism activities are all sources of empowerment and fulfillment for many people. Herbal medicine also helps people feel more in control of their healthcare decisions by giving them the freedom to select natural, plant-based treatments that suit their tastes, values, and beliefs.

Modern herbal medicine still faces difficulties and debates despite its increasing acceptability and popularity, especially in the areas of safety, quality assurance, and regulation. Herbal medicines are frequently marketed as dietary supplements. They are subject to less strict restrictions and quality control requirements than pharmaceutical pharmaceuticals, which must pass extensive testing and regulatory scrutiny prior to being licensed for sale. Inconsistencies in product potency, purity, and quality can result from this lack of oversight, and there may also be safety issues with contaminants, adulterants, and drug interactions. Furthermore, worries regarding false information, mislabeling, and inflated health claims, as well as the possibility of injury if used incorrectly or inappropriately, have arisen due to the extensive availability of herbal supplements and natural health products.

In summary, the emergence of contemporary herbal medicine is a reflection of the increased awareness of the therapeutic potential of medicinal plants as well as the importance of conventional medical methods in fostering health and well-being. Many people seeking alternatives to conventional therapies find that herbal therapy offers a natural, holistic approach to health in an era where pharmaceutical pill limitations and side effects are becoming more widely known. Modern herbal medicine is set to become more and more integrated into healthcare systems globally, bolstered by scientific research, consumer demand, and a growing interest in holistic health and self-care. Herbal medicine gives hope for a healthier, more sustainable future for people and the environment as we continue to investigate the possibilities of medicinal plants and combine traditional knowledge with modern science.

Exploring Plant Compounds with Antiviral Potential

The health of people is seriously threatened by viruses, which can cause a variety of infectious diseases that can result in morbidity, mortality, and worldwide pandemics. While antiviral medications and vaccines are valuable tools for treating and preventing viral infections, the rise of drug-resistant viruses and the limited effectiveness of current therapies highlight the need for novel therapeutic strategies. In recent times, there has been an increased focus on investigating the antiviral properties of plant compounds due to the abundance of bioactive molecules with diverse pharmacological activity found in natural products. Numerous secondary metabolites that are produced by plants, such as flavonoids, terpenoids, alkaloids, and phenolic chemicals, have been demonstrated to have antiviral activity against a range of human infections. Researchers are finding new antiviral drugs by utilizing nature's pharmacy, which has the potential to transform the way viral illnesses are treated and lessen the prevalence of viral diseases worldwide.

A comprehensive family of phytochemicals found in fruits, vegetables, herbs, and spices, polyphenols are one of the most promising groups of plant molecules with potential antiviral properties. Antioxidant and anti-inflammatory qualities, immune function modulation, and viral replication inhibition are among the well-known attributes of polyphenols. For instance, studies have demonstrated the antiviral solid activity of flavonoids like quercetin, resveratrol, and epigallocatechin gallate (EGCG) against a variety of viruses, such as the influenza virus, herpes simplex virus (HSV), HIV, and also severe acute respiratory syndrome coronavirus 2 (SARS-CoV-2). These substances modulate host cell signaling pathways involved in immune response as well as inflammation, as well as impede virus entrance, replication, and gene expression, among other mechanisms by which they exert their antiviral effects.

Alkaloids are another class of plant compounds that show promise as antiviral agents alongside polyphenols. Many medicinal plants include nitrogen-containing chemicals called alkaloids, which have long been employed for their therapeutic benefits. Potent inhibitors of viral replication have been found for a number of alkaloids, such as morphine, sanguinarine, and berberine. The antiviral activity of these compounds has been proven against several viruses, such as the hepatitis C virus (HCV), respiratory syncytial virus (RSV), and influenza virus. Alkaloids work against viruses by influencing host cell reactions to infection and by focusing on different phases of the virus life cycle, including protein synthesis, adhesion, and entrance.

Antiviral solid activity against a range of human infections is also exhibited by terpenoids, a varied class of hydrocarbons present in resinous exudates of plants and essential oils. Terpenoids exhibit a multitude of biological actions, such as immunomodulatory, antibacterial, and anti-inflammatory properties, as well as the inhibition of viral enzymes and disruption of viral replication. Compounds like eucalyptol, carvacrol, and thymol, for instance, have been demonstrated to have antiviral activity against human papillomavirus (HPV), herpes simplex virus (HSV), and respiratory viruses including influenza as well as respiratory syncytial virus (RSV). Terpenoids work against viruses by rupturing the integrity of the viral envelope, preventing viral entry and fusion, and interfering with the expression of viral genes and reproduction.

Many fruits, vegetables, and medicinal plants include a class of polyphenolic chemicals called flavonoids, which have garnered interest due to their possible antiviral capabilities. In addition to their capacity to prevent viral replication and lessen viral pathogenicity, flavonoids are widely recognized for their anti-inflammatory, immunomodulatory, and antioxidant properties. Examples of substances that have been demonstrated to provide antiviral action against various viruses include the herpes simplex virus (HSV), hepatitis C virus (HCV), influenza virus, and human immunodeficiency virus (HIV). These substances include hesperidin, naringenin, and quercetin. Flavonoids produce antiviral effects by interfering with the viral life cycle at different points, such as attachment, entrance, replication, and gene expression, and by modifying host cell signaling pathways linked to inflammation and the immune system.

In conclusion, it is essential to acknowledge that plant-based chemicals possess an abundance of bioactive molecules that exhibit diverse pharmacological properties, such as potent antiviral activity against a range of human illnesses. Scientists are finding novel therapeutic compounds through the investigation of plant chemicals' antiviral qualities, which could revolutionize the treatment of viral infections and reduce the incidence of viral diseases globally. Plant substances that show promise as antiviral agents include flavonoids, alkaloids, terpenoids, and polyphenols. Research is still being done to find new bioactive compounds with antiviral solid effects. The future is bright for the creation of secure, efficient, and reasonably priced herbal treatments for the avoidance and management of viral infections as long as we keep tapping into the power of nature's pharmacy.

CHAPTER III

Novel Herbal Antiviral Compounds

Cutting-Edge Research on Plant-Based Therapeutics

The demand for novel therapies for complicated diseases and the increasing awareness of the therapeutic potential of medicinal plants has led to a recent boom in interest in and funding for state-of-the-art research on plant-based medicines. Because plants have long been a rich source of bioactive compounds with a range of pharmacological properties, scientific developments have made it possible for researchers to explore and use the therapeutic potential of these natural products in ways that were before unattainable. Cutting-edge research on plant-based therapeutics is reshaping healthcare and agriculture, offering new hope for enhancing human health and well-being while promoting environmental sustainability and biodiversity conservation. This research is affecting everything from drug discovery and development to personalized medicine and precision agriculture.

Drug discovery and development is one of the most fascinating areas of plant-based therapeutics research, where researchers are using nature's pharmacy to find new chemicals with therapeutic promise. Technological advancements in analytical techniques, such as bioinformatics, metabolomics, and high-throughput screening, are making it easier to quickly identify and characterize the bioactive compounds found in medicinal plants and to clarify their mechanisms of action and potential therapeutic applications. Furthermore, scientists are now able to genetically modify plants to generate high-value pharmaceutical molecules, including immunomodulators, anticancer medications, and antibacterial agents, in enormous quantities and at a lower cost because of developments in synthetic biology and genetic engineering. These developments are transforming the process of finding new drugs and increasing the number of therapeutic molecules that patients and healthcare professionals may access.

Personalized medicine is another field of cutting-edge research in plant-based medicine. Here, researchers are using precision and genomic medicine techniques to customize treatments for specific patients according to their genetic composition, way of life, and surroundings. Researchers are learning more about how genetic variants affect drug response and disease risk, as well as how to discover biomarkers for predicting treatment results and directing therapeutic decisions by combining genomic data with clinical information. Additionally, pharmacogenomics breakthroughs are making it possible for researchers to pinpoint genetic variants that influence therapeutic efficacy, toxicity, and metabolism; this allows for the best possible drug selection and dosage for each patient. Because they provide a wide range of bioactive compounds that have the ability to target particular biochemical pathways and disease processes, as well as to alter the immune system and microbiota, plant-based treatments are essential to personalized medicine.

Advanced research in plant-based therapies is propelling innovation not only in personalized medicine and drug discovery but also in agriculture and environmental conservation. Through the application of genetic engineering and plant biotechnology, scientists are creating crops that are more environmentally friendly, have more nutritional content, have higher yields, and also are more resistant to pests and diseases. For instance, biofortified crops like iron- and zinc-fortified beans can help prevent malnutrition and enhance public health. In contrast, genetically modified crops like golden rice, fortified with beta-carotene, have the potential to address the widespread vitamin A deficiency in developing nations. Furthermore, developments in sustainable agriculture and agroecology are encouraging the growth of traditional crops and medicinal plants with ecological and cultural value. This supports local livelihoods, conserves biodiversity, and preserves traditional knowledge.

Plant-based therapies have great promise, but there are still a number of obstacles and opportunities to be addressed. The need to close the knowledge gap between traditional medicine and contemporary research and guarantee that all communities have fair access to the advantages of plant-based therapy is one of the significant problems. Indigenous peoples and traditional healers have long relied on medicinal plants to meet their healthcare needs, and their knowledge and experience are priceless assets for the research and development of new drugs. Furthermore, in order to preserve biodiversity, cultural legacy, and also traditional knowledge, the conservation and sustainable use of medicinal plants necessitate careful management and cooperation between scientists, policymakers, and local populations.

The requirement for thorough scientific investigation and evidence-based medicine to substantiate the security, effectiveness, and caliber of plant-based medications is another difficulty. The therapeutic benefits and methods of action of many medicinal plants, which have been utilized for centuries in traditional medical systems, sometimes need to be better understood and better recorded. In addition, inconsistent practices in the gathering, extraction, and formulation of plants can result in variations in the quality, potency, and purity of the final product, as well as safety issues with impurities, adulterants, and drug interactions. Therefore, to guarantee the safety and effectiveness of plant-based medications as well as to solve issues with quality control, standardization, and labeling, there is a need for thorough clinical trials and regulatory oversight.

In summary, state-of-the-art research on plant-based medicines is transforming agriculture and healthcare in the future by providing fresh chances to enhance human health and well-being and support environmental sustainability and biodiversity preservation. The fields of drug research, customized medicine, and sustainable agriculture are transforming healthcare and agriculture by utilizing nature's pharmacy to solve some of the most urgent problems confronting humankind. The therapeutic potential of medicinal plants is being unlocked by researchers by fusing traditional knowledge with contemporary science and technology, opening the door to a more sustainable and healthy future for both humans and the environment.

Bioactive Molecules with Antiviral Activity

A complex class of infectious organisms, viruses can cause anything from the ordinary cold to more serious conditions like HIV/AIDS, COVID-19, and influenza. As such, they represent severe hazards to human health. There is a pressing need for novel and efficient medicines to fight viral infections due to the rise of drug-resistant viruses and the shortcomings of current antiviral therapy. Investigating bioactive molecules with antiviral activity— naturally occurring substances present in plants, marine life, and microbes that can impede viral attachment, replication, entrance, and other phases of the viral life cycle—is one strategy that shows promise. The increasing worldwide burden of viral infections could be addressed with the help of these bioactive compounds, which provide a wealth of potential treatments.

Polyphenols are a broad family of phytochemicals that are present in fruits, vegetables, nuts, seeds, and plant-based beverages, including tea, coffee, and wine. They have strong antiviral properties. In addition to their capacity to prevent viral replication and lower viral load, polyphenols are well-known for their anti-inflammatory, immunomodulatory, and antioxidant qualities. For instance, studies have demonstrated the antiviral activity of flavonoids like quercetin, epigallocatechin gallate (EGCG), and catechins against a variety of viruses, such as the influenza virus, herpes simplex virus (HSV), respiratory syncytial virus (RSV), and human immunodeficiency virus (HIV). These flavonoids work against viruses by disrupting their attachment, entrance, and fusion phases, as well as by modifying host cell signaling pathways that are linked to inflammation and the immune system.

Alkaloids, nitrogen-containing chemicals present in many medicinal plants and fungi that have been traditionally employed for their therapeutic effects, are another family of bioactive molecules having antiviral activity. Alkaloids have potent antiviral activity against a spectrum of human infections in addition to their broad range of therapeutic activities, which include antibacterial, anti-inflammatory, and anticancer properties. For instance, it has been demonstrated that the benzylisoquinoline alkaloid berberine, which is present in plants including barberry and goldenseal, has antiviral properties against the human papillomavirus, hepatitis D virus, and influenza virus (HPV). Berberine works against viruses by reducing their ability to replicate and produce genes, as well as by influencing how host cells react to an infection.

Terpenoids are a broad class of hydrocarbons that are present in resinous plant exudates and essential oils. They have strong antiviral properties that can combat a range of human infections. Terpenoids are recognized for their capacity to impede viral enzymes and interfere with viral replication in addition to their antibacterial, anti-inflammatory, and immunomodulatory qualities. It has been demonstrated, for instance, that substances like eucalyptol, carvacrol, and thymol, which are present in plants like eucalyptus, oregano, and thyme, have antiviral properties against human papillomavirus (HPV), herpes simplex virus (HSV), and respiratory viruses like influenza and respiratory syncytial virus (RSV). By compromising the integrity of the viral envelope, preventing viral entrance and fusion, and interfering with viral replication and gene expression, these terpenoids achieve their antiviral actions.

Other bioactive compounds having antiviral activity include peptides, lipids, polysaccharides, and small molecules derived from microorganisms, natural sources, and marine species, in addition to polyphenols, alkaloids, and terpenoids. For instance, it has been demonstrated that peptides derived from marine sources, such as defensins and piscidins, have potent antiviral activity against a range of human infections, including both enveloped and non-enveloped viruses. Viral membrane integrity is disrupted, viral entrance and fusion are prevented, and host cell responses to infection are modulated by these peptides in order to achieve their antiviral effects. Similar to this, it has been demonstrated that lipids derived from marine sources, including omega-3 fatty acids, have antiviral properties against hepatitis C and HIV, as well as respiratory viruses like influenza and respiratory syncytial virus (RSV) (HCV). These lipids impede viral replication and gene expression, as well as alter host cell signaling pathways connected to inflammation and immunological response in order to produce their antiviral effects.

In summary, bioactive compounds possessing antiviral properties provide a plethora of promising treatments that may contribute to mitigating the increasing worldwide prevalence of viral illnesses. As potent inhibitors of viral replication, attachment, entry, and also other stages of the viral life cycle, polyphenols, alkaloids, terpenoids, peptides, lipids, polysaccharides, and other bioactive compounds derived from plants, marine animals, and microorganisms have shown promise. Researchers are discovering innovative therapies that have the potential to transform the treatment of viral infections and enhance human health and well-being by investigating the antiviral activity of these natural molecules. There is a lot of hope for the creation of safe, efficient, and reasonably priced antiviral drugs derived from nature's pharmacy as we continue to understand the nuances of viral pathogenesis and host-virus interactions.

Harnessing Nature's Arsenal against Viral Infections

Viruses are common pathogens that can cause a variety of infectious diseases that can result in morbidity, mortality, and worldwide pandemics. As such, they represent severe risks to human health. Viral infections continue to be a problem for global healthcare systems and public health initiatives, ranging from the common cold to more severe conditions like influenza, HIV/AIDS, and COVID-19. The rise of drug-resistant viruses and the shortcomings of current treatments underline the need for novel therapeutic methods, even while vaccinations and antiviral medications are valuable tools for treating and preventing viral infections. Using the vast array of bioactive chemicals that are present in plants, marine life, and microbes that have evolved to fend against viral infections is one effective tactic for combating viral infections.

It has long been known that plants are an essential source of bioactive substances with a variety of pharmacological characteristics, such as antiviral solid activity. All around the world, traditional medical systems rely heavily on medicinal herbs, which have long been used to treat a variety of illnesses, including viral infections. Researchers have found a number of bioactive compounds that block viral multiplication, attachment, entrance, and other stages of the viral life cycle by examining the antiviral potential of medicinal plants. For instance, it has been demonstrated that terpenoids like thymol, alkaloids like berberine, and polyphenols like flavonoids all have antiviral solid effects against a range of human infections. These organic substances present encouraging avenues for the creation of novel antiviral medications and treatments that may aid in the fight against viral infections and lessen the prevalence of viral illnesses worldwide.

Marine life is another abundant source of bioactive compounds with antiviral properties, in addition to plants. In order to survive in harsh marine settings, marine species have developed unique defensive mechanisms. One such mechanism is the synthesis of bioactive chemicals that provide protection against viruses and other microbial diseases. By examining the antiviral potential of compounds derived from marine sources, researchers have found a plethora of natural molecules with strong antiviral activity against a variety of human illnesses. For instance, it has been demonstrated that peptides derived from marine sources, such as ascidians and defensins, had antiviral solid properties against both enclosed and non-enveloped viruses, such as the hepatitis C virus, HIV, and influenza virus. Similarly, it has been demonstrated that lipids derived from marine sources, including omega-3 fatty acids, have antiviral properties against respiratory viruses like respiratory syncytial virus and influenza virus (RSV). These chemicals originating from marine sources have intriguing opportunities for the creation of novel antiviral medications and treatments that may aid in the fight against viral infections and enhance human health.

In addition to producing bioactive compounds with antiviral action, microorganisms—including bacteria, fungi, and viruses—also have the capacity to be used therapeutically. For instance, bacteria-infecting viruses called bacteriophages generate endolysins, which are enzymes that can damage bacterial cell walls. This could provide a unique therapeutic option for bacterial infections, which are frequently linked to viral infections. Comparably, some fungi generate bioactive substances such as polysaccharides and beta-glucans that have been demonstrated to have antiviral and immunomodulatory properties against a range of human infections. Through investigating the antiviral capabilities of microorganisms and their byproducts, scientists are finding new directions for the creation of cutting-edge antiviral medications and treatments that may aid in the fight against viral infections and lessen the prevalence of viral illnesses worldwide.

In conclusion, a multitude of bioactive compounds with antiviral solid activity found in nature can potentially be used for medicinal applications. There are countless substances in the natural world, ranging from bacteria to plants and marine life, that have developed defenses against viral infections. Researchers are finding new directions for the creation of cutting-edge antiviral medications and treatments that may aid in the fight against viral infections and enhance human health by investigating the antiviral potential of these natural substances. There is a lot of hope for the creation of safe, efficient, and reasonably priced antiviral drugs derived from nature's pharmacy as we continue to understand the nuances of viral pathogenesis and host-virus interactions.

CHAPTER IV

Herbal Antivirals: Mechanisms of Action

Dissecting the Molecular Targets of Herbal Compounds

For ages, people from many cultures have used herbal medicine as a primary or supplemental means of treating a wide range of illnesses. The diverse variety of bioactive chemicals found in medicinal plants is responsible for the therapeutic efficacy of these medicines. These compounds work by interacting with specific molecular targets within the body. Thanks to developments in molecular biology, pharmacology, and bioinformatics, there has been an increasing amount of interest in analyzing the molecular targets of herbal substances in recent years. Researchers hope to get a better understanding of herbal compounds' therapeutic benefits, maximize their application in clinical practice, and identify new drug targets for the creation of innovative treatments by clarifying the molecular mechanisms of action of these compounds.

Using high-throughput screening tests to find plausible targets and mechanisms of action is one method for analyzing the molecular targets of herbal medicines. With the aid of these assays, scientists may quickly sort through vast libraries of herbal compounds in order to find those with the highest affinity and specificity against a variety of biological targets, including enzymes, receptors, and signaling cascades. Researchers can learn more about the structural characteristics of herbal compounds and how they interact with target proteins by combining high-throughput screening with computer modeling and bioinformatics analysis. This allows for the rational creation and optimization of drugs. Furthermore, the three-dimensional structures of herbal compounds and their target proteins have been clarified thanks to advancements in structural biology techniques like nuclear magnetic resonance (NMR) spectroscopy and X-ray crystallography. These discoveries have provided atomic-level insights into the binding interactions and mechanisms of action of these compounds.

Analyzing the global impacts of herbal remedies on biological systems through the application of omics technologies, such as transcriptomics, proteomics, metabolomics, and genomes, is another method for analyzing the molecular targets of herbal substances. With the aid of these tools, researchers may gain a thorough understanding of the molecular consequences of herbal therapies by profiling changes in protein abundance, gene expression, and metabolite levels. Researchers can determine critical pathways and networks that herbal substances target, as well as possible biomarkers of treatment response or side effects, by combining omics data with computer modeling and systems biology techniques. Furthermore, developments in pharmacogenomics and network pharmacology are opening the door for precision medicine methods in herbal medicine by allowing researchers to tailor herbal remedies based on unique genetic variations and disease phenotypes, as well as forecast drug-target interactions.

To determine the molecular targets of herbal medicines, researchers are using empirical data and traditional knowledge in addition to experimental and computational methodologies. Traditional medical systems have long depended on observations of the therapeutic benefits of medicinal plants and herbal remedies in treating a variety of health disorders. Ayurveda, traditional herbalism, and Traditional Chinese Medicine (TCM) are a few of these systems. Researchers can find similarities and patterns in the application of herbal compounds in various cultures and traditions, as well as clarify their mechanisms of action based on traditional indications and therapeutic effects, by methodically recording and cataloging traditional knowledge. Furthermore, research on ethnobotany and ethnopharmacology is yielding critical new understandings of the therapeutic qualities of plants utilized by native American tribes and nearby communities, as well as their possible molecular targets and modes of action.

The complexity and diversity of bioactive chemicals found in medicinal plants, along with their pleiotropic effects on many targets and pathways inside the body, create a problem in identifying the molecular targets of herbal compounds. Unlike single-target medications, which frequently have a strong affinity and selectivity for a single molecular target, herbal medicines may have many modes of action, including synergistic interactions between various bioactive components. Further confounding their pharmacological effects and molecular targets are the considerable variations in the bioavailability and pharmacokinetics of herbal substances based on patient characteristics, dosage, method of administration, and formulation. Therefore, to thoroughly analyze the molecular targets of herbal substances and clarify their modes of action in health and disease, interdisciplinary techniques integrating experimental, computational, and traditional methods are required.

Conclusively, analyzing the molecular targets of herbal substances is an intricate and multidisciplinary undertaking with significant potential to enhance our comprehension of their therapeutic impacts and methods of action. Researchers are discovering new pharmacological targets for the creation of innovative treatments and learning more about the molecular underpinnings of herbal medicine by fusing experimental, computational, and traditional methods. Furthermore, customized approaches to herbal medicine based on unique genetic variants and disease phenotypes are becoming possible thanks to developments in omics technology, network pharmacology, and precision medicine. The future is bright for the creation of secure, efficient, and customized herbal remedies for a variety of medical issues as we continue to decipher the mysteries of herbal medicine and harness the power of nature's pharmacy.

Modulating Viral Entry, Replication, and Assembly

Viruses are challenging targets for therapeutic intervention because they are intracellular parasites that depend on host cells for replication and propagation. Nevertheless, by focusing on crucial stages of the viral life cycle, like viral entrance, replication, and assembly, scientists have discovered a number of methods for adjusting viral infections and creating antiviral treatments. Determining possible therapeutic targets and creating potent antiviral tactics require an understanding of the molecular mechanisms underpinning viral entrance, replication, and assembly. Researchers want to create new treatments that can stop viral infections, slow down viral replication, and stop the spread of viral diseases by breaking down these processes at the molecular level.

The adherence of viral particles to host cell receptors, internalization, and release of the viral DNA into the host cell comprise the first stage of the viral life cycle. Since it can prevent the virus from infecting and propagating within a host, antiviral medication that targets viral entry is an attractive treatment option. The creation of entrance inhibitors that specifically target host cell receptors or viral attachment proteins is one method of controlling viral entry. Fusion inhibitors, including enfuvirtide and maraviroc, impede the merging of viral and cellular membranes by selectively binding to either the host cell's chemokine receptors or the viral envelope proteins. Similar to this, attachment inhibitors like lectins and glycan-binding proteins can stop viruses from attaching to glycans on host cell surfaces, which stops viruses from infecting cells and spreading. Researchers want to create treatments that can stop the propagation of viral pathogens within the host and stop infection in its tracks by focusing on viral entrance.

The process by which virus genomes are duplicated and viral proteins are made in host cells results in the creation of new virus particles, known as viral replication. Another crucial tactic for antiviral therapy is to target viral replication, which can stop the creation of infectious virions and restrict viral dissemination inside the host. The creation of nucleoside analogs and polymerase inhibitors that specifically target viral RNA or DNA polymerases involved in viral genome replication is one method of regulating viral replication. For instance, by competing with natural nucleoside substrates, medications like tenofovir and acyclovir inhibit viral DNA polymerases, preventing the manufacture and replication of viral DNA. Viral proteases that are involved in the processing and maturation of viral proteins can be inhibited by protease inhibitors like lopinavir and ritonavir. This can effectively stop the formation of infectious virions. Researchers hope to create treatments that can stop the synthesis of new viral particles and restrict the spread of the virus inside the host by focusing on viral replication.

The packing of viral genomes and proteins into new viral particles, followed by the budding and discharge of virions from host cells, constitutes the final stage of the viral life cycle. Antiviral therapy that targets viral assembly shows promise since it can stop the creation of infectious virions and stop the virus from spreading inside the host. The creation of assembly inhibitors that target host cell components or viral structural proteins involved in viral particle production is one method of modifying viral assembly. For instance, medications like zanamivir and oseltamivir prevent the release of fresh viral particles from infected cells, inhibiting viral neuraminidases and restricting the transmission of the virus within the host. Similarly, medications that inhibit the formation of infectious virions, such as ribavirin and interferons, can alter host cell components involved in viral assembly and release. Researchers hope to create treatments that can stop the creation of new viral particles and restrict the spread of the virus inside the host by focusing on viral assembly.

In conclusion, as it can stop the propagation of the virus within the host, prevent infection from starting, and impede viral reproduction, regulating viral entry, assembly, and replication offers a viable approach to antiviral therapy. Researchers are able to build innovative therapies that can interrupt critical steps in the viral life cycle and find prospective drug targets by comprehending the molecular mechanics underlying these activities.

There are several ways to modify viral infections and create efficient antiviral treatments, ranging from entry inhibitors that prevent viral attachment and fusion to replication inhibitors that target viral polymerases and proteases and assembly inhibitors that prevent viral particle formation and release. The development of safe, efficient, and tailored antiviral medicines that can combat a broad spectrum of viral infections and enhance human health is looking very promising as scientists continue to untangle the intricate web of viral pathogenesis and host-virus interactions.

Synergy and Combinatorial Approaches in Herbal Therapeutics

For thousands of years, people from many cultures have used herbal medicine as a primary or supplemental treatment for a wide range of illnesses. The complex mixture of bioactive chemicals found in medicinal plants, which can have synergistic effects when used in combination, is frequently credited with the therapeutic success of herbal treatments. When two or more chemicals work together to have a higher effect than the sum of their separate effects, a phenomenon known as synergy occurs that improves treatment outcomes. Combinatorial methods address several pathways or mechanisms implicated in disease pathogenesis by using multiple herbal ingredients or formulations in a sequential or simultaneous manner. Researchers hope to maximize the therapeutic efficiency of herbal medicines and enhance patient outcomes by utilizing the complimentary effects of many herbs as well as the synergistic interactions between various bioactive components.

The capacity of synergy and combinatorial techniques in herbal therapies to target several pathways or mechanisms involved in the etiology of disease is one of their main advantages. Numerous illnesses are intricate and multifaceted, entailing the disruption of various biological pathways and activities. In comparison to single-target therapies, mixtures of herbal substances that target many elements of disease pathophysiology can help researchers overcome drug resistance and achieve tremendous therapeutic success. Combinatorial methods comprising several herbal substances with anticancer effects, for instance, can target tumor cells through a variety of pathways, including immune system regulation, blockage of angiogenesis, and activation of apoptosis. Analogously, in the management of infectious disorders, the body's defenses against pathogens and ability to halt disease development can be strengthened by the synergistic interactions of herbal substances with antiviral, antibacterial, and immunomodulatory qualities.

Reducing side effects and toxicity linked to high doses of single substances is another benefit of synergy and combinatorial techniques in herbal therapies. When administered in large quantities, many herbal substances have limited therapeutic windows and can have deleterious effects that are dependent on dosage.

Researchers can produce therapeutic results at lower dosages of each herbal compound, lowering the risk of side effects and toxicity by combining substances that target distinct areas of disease etiology. Furthermore, the synergistic interactions among the constituents of herbal medicines might augment their therapeutic efficacy, so permitting the use of lower doses without sacrificing efficacy. For instance, combinatorial techniques using several herbal substances with anti-inflammatory and analgesic qualities can reduce pain and inflammation with fewer side effects than single-target therapy in the treatment of inflammatory disorders like rheumatoid arthritis.

Herbal treatments' synergistic and combinatorial techniques provide advantages for precision dosing and customized therapy in addition to their therapeutic effects. Since each person is different, the way they respond to herbal medicines differs based on lifestyle choices, genetics, and environmental exposures.

Researchers can maximize therapeutic success and reduce the chance of side effects by customizing herbal formulations to the unique qualities of each patient and the disease phenotype. Furthermore, researchers are now able to discover genetic differences that impact medication response and metabolism thanks to advancements in pharmacogenomics and precision medicine. This enables the creation of customized dosage regimens based on individual genetic profiles.
Researchers hope to create safer, more precise, and more

effective herbal medicines that can enhance patient outcomes and quality of life by fusing combinatorial and synergistic techniques with personalized medicine.

Synergy and combinatorial techniques in herbal medicines have advantages, but they also have drawbacks. The intricacy and diversity of herbal formulations, which can include hundreds or even thousands of bioactive components with various pharmacological characteristics, is one of the primary obstacles. It can be challenging to choose the best herbal ingredient combination and dosage schedule; this requires extensive testing in clinical settings. Furthermore, there can be significant variations in the strength, purity, and efficacy of herbal products due to a need for more standardization and also quality control. To guarantee the security and effectiveness of herbal products, standardized procedures for the preparation, extraction, and formulation of herbal medicines are therefore required, along with strict quality control procedures.

To sum up, herbal treatments' synergistic and combinatorial techniques present viable methods for enhancing the therapeutic effectiveness of herbal remedies and enhancing patient outcomes. The goal of this research is to target multiple pathways or mechanisms involved in disease pathogenesis, reduce adverse effects and toxicity, and personalize dosing regimens based on unique patient characteristics by utilizing the synergistic interactions between different bioactive compounds and the complementary effects of multiple herbs. While standardization of formulations, quality assurance, and clinical testing continue to be obstacles, combinatorial methods, and synergy have significant potential benefits in herbal therapies. There is a lot of hope for the creation of safer, more potent, and more individualized herbal therapies in the future as we work to understand the complexities of herbal medicine and investigate the possibility of synergistic interactions between herbal compounds.

CHAPTER V

Herbs of Interest: Antiviral Powerhouses

Spotlight on Promising Herbal Species

For thousands of years, herbal medicine has been a vital component of human healthcare, providing all-natural cures for a variety of illnesses. Many civilizations have used medicinal plants historically to treat ailments, reduce symptoms, and enhance general health. Concerns regarding the efficacy and safety of traditional medicines, along with rising awareness of the therapeutic potential of medicinal plants, have led to a renaissance of interest in herbal therapy in recent years. These days, medical professionals and researchers are focusing on promising plant species to learn more about their therapeutic qualities, modes of action, and prospective uses in contemporary medicine.

Curcuma longa, or turmeric, is an herbal species that has shown promise and has attracted attention recently. The flowering plant turmeric is indigenous to South Asia, where it has been utilized for ages in traditional medical systems, including Traditional Chinese Medicine (TCM) and Ayurveda. It has been demonstrated that curcumin, the main ingredient in turmeric, has potent anti-inflammatory, antioxidant, and anticancer effects.

Research has indicated that curcumin has the ability to impede the function of enzymes that promote inflammation, adjust immunological responses, and impede the development and dissemination of cancerous cells. Furthermore, curcumin has been shown to lessen the side effects of traditional cancer therapies like radiation and chemotherapy while increasing their effectiveness. As a result, studies are being conducted on turmeric and curcumin as possible therapies for a range of illnesses, including cancer, diabetes, cardiovascular disease, and arthritis.

Indian ginseng, winter cherry, or ashwagandha (Withania somnifera) is another herb that shows promise. Native to India and North Africa, ashwagandha is a tiny shrub that has been utilized for thousands of years in ancient medical systems like Ayurveda and Unani therapy. Withanolides, a class of bioactive chemicals found in the root of the ashwagandha plant, have been demonstrated to have immunomodulatory, adaptogenic, and anti-stress effects. Research has shown that ashwagandha extracts help strengthen the immune system, lessen stress and anxiety, and improve cognitive and physical performance. Additionally, studies have shown that ashwagandha has neuroprotective and anti-inflammatory properties, which suggests that it may be used to treat diseases including Parkinson's, Alzheimer's, and arthritis. As a result, ashwagandha is becoming more well-liked as a home cure for common health issues like stress and exhaustion.

Another herbal species that has gained popularity due to its possible health advantages is ginkgo biloba. A rare kind of tree endemic to China, ginkgo biloba has been grown there for thousands of years due to its therapeutic benefits. Bioactive substances found in ginkgo tree leaves, such as terpenoids and flavonoids, have been demonstrated to have neuroprotective, anti-inflammatory, and antioxidant qualities. Ginkgo biloba extracts have been shown in studies to protect against age-related improved memory, cognitive decline, concentration, and improved cognitive performance. In addition, ginkgo biloba has been demonstrated to lessen inflammation, enhance blood flow, and guard against oxidative stress, suggesting that it may be used as a treatment for ailments like dementia, Alzheimer's disease, and cardiovascular disease. Ginkgo biloba is so frequently used as a home treatment for memory loss, cognitive decline, and other health issues associated with aging.

Purple coneflower, or Echinacea purpurea, is another herbaceous species that has become well-known for its possible immune-stimulating abilities. Native Americans have been using the perennial herb echinacea for millennia to treat wounds, infections, and other conditions. It is native to North America. Bioactive substances like alkamides, polysaccharides, and flavonoids, which have been demonstrated to have immunomodulatory, anti-inflammatory, and antibacterial qualities, are found in the roots, leaves, and flowers of the echinacea plant. Research has indicated that echinacea extracts have the ability to incite immune cell activity, augment the generation of antibodies, and mitigate the intensity and length of colds and other respiratory diseases. Additionally, echinacea has been shown to have anti-inflammatory and antioxidant properties, which suggests that it may be used as a treatment for ailments like autoimmune illnesses, allergies, and asthma. Echinacea is, therefore, frequently used as a home medicine to increase immunity and ward against diseases.

To sum up, there are a lot of intriguing species of herbs that may have medicinal and health benefits. These herbal treatments, which include ginkgo biloba, echinacea, turmeric, and ashwagandha, have been utilized for millennia in traditional medical systems and are now becoming more well-known for their therapeutic qualities in contemporary healthcare. Though further investigation is necessary to completely comprehend their modes of action, effectiveness, and safety, these plant species have enormous potential as all-natural treatments for a variety of illnesses. Researchers and medical professionals are looking into novel approaches to harness the therapeutic potential of medicinal plants and incorporate them into evidence-based healthcare procedures as interest in herbal medicine grows. Herbal medicine has the potential to significantly contribute to the promotion of health and well-being as well as the enhancement of people's quality of life worldwide with more research and innovation.

Traditional Uses and Contemporary Validation

People have always looked to nature for cures and health-promoting products to relieve their diseases. For thousands of years, traditional medical systems have been an integral part of healthcare, drawing on indigenous knowledge and cultural customs. From Indigenous healing practices in the Americas to African traditional medicine, and from Ayurveda in India to Traditional Chinese Medicine (TCM) in China, every culture has developed its own methods for diagnosing and treating disease with locally accessible plants, minerals, and other natural substances. Traditional medicine practitioners and supporters have long held the belief that their methods work, yet in modern healthcare systems, their legitimacy and acceptability are sometimes greeted with suspicion and examination. Nonetheless, there has been a deliberate attempt in recent years to verify the safety and effectiveness of conventional medicine through scientific study and clinical trials, as well as a rising appreciation of its benefits.

Traditional medicine's all-encompassing approach to health and wellness is among its most appealing features. The interconnection of the body, mind, and spirit is emphasized by traditional medical systems, in contrast to Western medicine, which frequently concentrates on treating specific symptoms or disorders. According to traditional medical practitioners, illness results from imbalances or interruptions in the body's equilibrium, which is maintained in a condition of harmony and balance during health. Therefore, in order to restore balance and enhance general well-being, traditional healing techniques frequently combine medical, psychological, and spiritual approaches. For instance, Ayurveda, the traditional Indian medical system, emphasizes lifestyle adjustments, dietary adjustments, herbal medicines, and yoga as ways to prevent and treat illness. It bases its tailored approach to health on each person's distinct constitution or dosha. Similarly, yin and yang are seen as opposing energies that must be in balance for health to exist. Traditional Chinese Medicine (TCM) employs qigong, herbal medicine, food therapy, and acupuncture to achieve this balance and support health.

Despite the fact that traditional medicine systems have been used for centuries and have a wealth of anecdotal evidence to support their usefulness, a lack of rigorous clinical trials and scientific data has frequently made it difficult for modern healthcare systems to embrace and validate these systems. Opponents of conventional medicine contend that a large number of traditional treatments are not supported by evidence-based protocols, standardized formulations, or quality control procedures, which makes it challenging to evaluate their efficacy, safety, and repeatability. Furthermore, empirical data, cultural values, and metaphysical ideas are frequently the foundation of traditional medical treatments, which may not conform to Western scientific paradigms or procedures. Because of this, some legislators and medical experts have been reluctant to include traditional medicine in mainstream healthcare systems without sufficient regulatory control and scientific proof.

The validation of traditional medicine's safety and efficacy by scientific research and clinical trials has garnered attention in recent times. Scholars worldwide are progressively focusing on conventional healing methods, investigating their therapeutic potential, mechanisms of action, and possible integration into contemporary healthcare. Researchers are gaining insights into the pharmacological properties of traditional remedies, identifying their active ingredients and mechanisms of action, and assessing their safety and efficacy in rigorous clinical trials by utilizing contemporary scientific methods and technologies, such as pharmacology, biochemistry, genomics, and clinical epidemiology. Furthermore, developments in ethnopharmacology, ethnobotany, and phytochemistry are allowing scientists to collect and record the therapeutic qualities of plants utilized in traditional medicine systems and to find novel bioactive substances with promising therapeutic applications.

Herbal medicine has drawn a lot of interest recently as one branch of traditional medicine. Many contemporary medications are derived from or inspired by plant-based substances, which have long been utilized as treatments for a variety of illnesses in traditional medical systems around the world. These days, scientists are delving into the pharmacological characteristics, active components, and mechanisms of action of medicinal plants utilized in traditional medicine in order to investigate their therapeutic potential. Researchers hope to find potential new medications for treating a variety of disorders by putting traditional herbal treatments through rigorous scientific analysis in order to validate their safety and efficacy. Herbs like ginger, garlic, and turmeric, for instance, have been demonstrated in tests to have strong anti-inflammatory, antioxidant, and antibacterial qualities. As a result, these herbs may be used to treat diseases, including cancer, arthritis, and cardiovascular disease. Herbs that have been shown to have adaptogenic, neuroprotective, and immunomodulatory properties include ginseng, ginkgo biloba, and ashwagandha. As a result, these plants may be used as remedies for autoimmune illnesses, stress, and cognitive decline.

Apart from herbal medicine, other conventional healing modalities, including massage therapy, acupuncture, and mind-body interventions, are also being investigated and verified by scientific research. For example, studies have demonstrated that acupuncture modifies immunological responses, regulates the autonomic nervous system, and increases the production of endorphins and also other neurotransmitters. As a result, it may be used as a treatment for a variety of illnesses, including chronic pain, anxiety, and depression. Likewise, massage therapy has been demonstrated to alleviate tense muscles, enhance blood flow, and encourage rest, indicating its promise as a remedy for musculoskeletal discomfort, problems associated with stress, and irregular sleep patterns. The practice of tai chi, yoga, and meditation are examples of mind-body treatments that have been demonstrated to improve mood, lower stress levels, and improve general well-being. They can also be used as adjuvant therapy for a range of illnesses, both physical and mental.

In conclusion, a wide range of time-tested healing techniques that have been handed down through the ages are available in traditional medicine. Traditional medicine practitioners and supporters have long held the belief that their methods work, yet in modern healthcare systems, their legitimacy and acceptability are sometimes greeted with suspicion and examination. Nonetheless, there has been a deliberate attempt in recent years to verify the safety and effectiveness of conventional medicine through scientific study and clinical trials, as well as a rising appreciation of its benefits. Through the use of contemporary scientific tools and techniques, scientists are learning more about the pharmacological characteristics of conventional treatments, pinpointing their active components and modes of action, and conducting thorough clinical trials to assess their efficacy and safety. Researchers, medical professionals, and policymakers are collaborating to incorporate traditional healing practices into evidence-based healthcare systems in response to the growing interest in traditional medicine. This is done to guarantee that patients have access to safe, efficient, and culturally relevant treatments for their health and well-being.

Cultivation, Extraction, and Standardization Challenges

Herbal medicine involves several complicated and unique challenges in the core areas of medicinal plant cultivation, extraction, and standardization. Throughout history, herbal medicine has been used by societies all over the world for thousands of years to promote health and treat illnesses. It is based on the medicinal qualities of plants. However, with the growing popularity of herbal remedies in the current era, it's critical to overcome the difficulties in growing, extracting, and standardizing medicinal plants in order to guarantee their quality, safety, and efficacy.

Many issues, such as genetic variability, sustainability concerns, and environmental circumstances, might make it challenging to cultivate therapeutic plants. For many medicinal plants to flourish and efficiently produce bioactive substances, particular environmental factors, such as soil type, climate, and altitude, are necessary.

Furthermore, attempts to cultivate medicinal plants sustainably are required due to the decrease of wild plant populations brought on by overexploitation and habitat destruction. Examples of sustainable agriculture practices that aim to lessen their adverse effects on the environment while preserving the long-term viability of populations of medicinal plants include wildcrafting, agroforestry, and organic farming. However, these approaches require careful planning, monitoring, and management in order to balance ecological, social, and economic issues.

Plant chemistry is complicated and diverse, which presents additional hurdles when extracting bioactive chemicals from medicinal plants. Alkaloids, flavonoids, terpenoids, and phenolic compounds are just a few of the many bioactive substances found in medicinal plants. Each has distinct chemical characteristics and physiological effects. To ensure the effective and selective extraction of target compounds while reducing the extraction of undesired elements, extraction methods need to be carefully chosen and refined. Depending on the characteristics of the target chemicals and the intended end product, standard extraction procedures include maceration, percolation, Soxhlet extraction, and supercritical fluid extraction. Each has advantages and disadvantages.

For customers to be sure of consistency, quality, and safety, herbal products must be standardized. Standardization entails creating criteria based on scientific principles and legal requirements for the identity, purity, potency, and composition of herbal items. However, because of differences in plant genetics, growing environments, and processing methods, uniformity can be difficult. The amount of bioactive chemicals in different cultivars of the same plant species may vary, and plant chemistry can also be influenced by changes in soil composition, climate, and cultivation techniques. Furthermore, processing methods, including extraction, grinding, and drying, might affect the amount and makeup of bioactive substances in herbal products.

Therefore, in order to assure consistency and potency, standardization efforts must take these issues into account and establish vital analytical methodologies and quality control systems.

Herbal medicine's production, extraction, and standardization issues need for a multidisciplinary strategy that integrates conventional wisdom with cutting-edge scientific tools and techniques. The development and implementation of sustainable farming strategies are vital to guarantee the long-term sustainability of medicinal plant populations while mitigating their influence on the environment. In order to reduce the amount of energy and solvents used and increase the yield and purity of bioactive chemicals, extraction techniques must be adjusted. It is imperative that standardization efforts be thorough and rigorous, accounting for differences in plant chemistry, growing environments, and processing methods.

Furthermore, in order to overcome the difficulties associated with cultivation, extraction, and standardization in herbal medicine, cooperation and coordination between researchers, farmers, manufacturers, regulators, and healthcare practitioners are crucial. Collaboratively, stakeholders can exchange best practices, resources, and expertise to guarantee the efficacy, safety, and quality of herbal products.

Furthermore, in order to handle new opportunities and problems in herbal medicine, continuous research, and innovation in cultivation strategies, extraction processes, and standardization procedures are required.

Finally, it should be noted that the crucial components of herbal medicine—cultivation, extraction, and standardization—present particular difficulties and complications. Vital standardization initiatives, efficient extraction techniques, and sustainable farming methods are necessary to guarantee the efficacy, safety, and caliber of herbal products. To tackle these obstacles, a multidisciplinary strategy, cooperation between relevant parties, and continuous investigation and creativity are necessary. Herbal medicine can still be a valuable tool for improving health and treating ailments in the modern era by addressing the issues with cultivation, extraction, and standardization.

CHAPTER VI

Clinical Applications of Herbal Antivirals

Integrative Medicine: Merging Tradition with Modernity

Integrative medicine, sometimes referred to as complementary and alternative medicine (CAM), is a method of treating patients that integrates established medical procedures with supplementary therapies and healing practices. Integrative medicine uses a wide range of healing approaches from around the globe to address the physical, emotional, and spiritual components of health and wellness. This method seeks to deliver individualized, holistic care that takes into account each patient's particular needs while acknowledging that a variety of factors, including genetics, lifestyle, environment, and sociocultural factors, can affect health and illness. Integrative medicine provides a complete and patient-centered approach to healthcare that prioritizes empowerment, cooperation, and self-care by fusing tradition with modernity.

Recognizing the value of ancient healing methods in promoting health and treating ailments lies at the core of integrative medicine. With thousands of years of history, traditional medical systems, including Ayurveda, Traditional Chinese Medicine (TCM), and Indigenous healing techniques, have been used to treat a broad spectrum of illnesses. In order to restore balance and enhance well-being, these systems highlight the connection between the body, mind, and spirit and use a range of therapies, such as energy healing, herbal medicine, acupuncture, massage therapy, and mind-body

techniques. In order to give patients a more thorough and all-encompassing approach to recovery, integrative medicine acknowledges the importance of these age-old healing techniques and works to incorporate them into contemporary healthcare systems.

Integrative medicine combines current medical procedures and technologies with ancient healing methods to give patients the best of both worlds. Conventional medical interventions, including medication, surgery, and medical equipment, have transformed healthcare and saved a great deal of lives. These treatments, however, may have drawbacks or side effects and frequently concentrate on treating symptoms rather than the fundamental causes of sickness. Integrative medicine aims to enhance traditional medical care by utilizing complementary therapies and practices that target the underlying causes of disease and facilitate physical, mental, and spiritual healing. Through the integration of modern and traditional medical practices, integrative medicine provides patients with a more customized and all-encompassing healthcare experience that takes into account their individual requirements, preferences, and objectives.

The value of patient and healthcare provider cooperation and partnership is one of integrative medicine's fundamental tenets. In integrated medicine, patients are encouraged to take an active role in managing their health, preventing illness, and making healthcare decisions. Together, patients and healthcare providers develop personalized treatment programs that address each patient's particular needs, preferences, and goals.

They act as mentors, instructors, and collaborators in the healing process. This cooperative approach gives patients the power to take charge of their own health and well-being and promotes mutual respect, trust, and communication between patients and doctors.

The emphasis on wellness and prevention is a critical component of integrative medicine. Integrative medicine emphasizes the need to form good lifestyle habits, such as appropriate diet, consistent exercise, stress management, and enough sleep. It acknowledges that sustaining health and preventing sickness are crucial components of healthcare. Integrative medicine seeks to maximize health and stop disease before it starts by addressing the underlying causes of illness and encouraging wellness on a physical, emotional, and spiritual level. Better health outcomes, lower healthcare costs, and an improvement in the standard of living for both individuals and communities can result from this proactive approach to healthcare.

Integrative medicine has numerous advantages, but it also has drawbacks. One issue is that some complementary therapies and practices need more scientific backing, which may make it challenging for medical professionals to advocate or prescribe these treatments confidently. Furthermore, some patients may not be able to obtain integrative medicine since it is not funded by healthcare systems or covered by insurance. In addition, people may face obstacles related to their culture, social standing, or financial situation when trying to get integrative treatment, especially in underprivileged areas. In order to address these issues and enhance access to care for everyone, more research, instruction, lobbying, and legislative changes are needed to support the integration of integrative medicine into traditional healthcare systems.

To sum up, integrative medicine provides a thorough, patient-centered approach to healthcare by fusing the best elements of modern and traditional medicine. Integrative medicine acknowledges the importance of conventional therapeutic methods while embracing the most recent developments in medical procedures and technological innovations. This method aims to address

the mental, emotional, and spiritual facets of health and wellness while placing a strong emphasis on empowerment, teamwork, and self-care. Integrative medicine is a significant and promising approach to healthcare in the modern world despite its difficulties and limitations. It could lead to better health outcomes, less expensive healthcare, and a higher standard of living.

Clinical Trials and Evidence-Based Practice

The foundation of evidence-based practice in healthcare is clinical trials, which offer essential insights into the efficacy, safety, and effectiveness of medical interventions and treatments. Clinical trials are intended to produce high-quality evidence that can guide healthcare decisions and enhance patient outcomes. They are conducted in compliance with strict scientific standards and ethical norms. Clinical trials are essential for expanding medical knowledge, guiding clinical practice, and determining public health policy because they methodically assess the advantages and disadvantages of medicinal interventions. The significance of clinical trials in evidence-based practice, the significant stages of clinical trial research, ethical issues in conducting clinical trials, the difficulties and constraints of clinical trial research, and the prospects for clinical trial methodology are all covered in this section.

The foundation of evidence-based practice in healthcare is the combination of patient preferences and values, professional competence, and the best available data from clinical research. Evidence from clinical trials is essential for guiding healthcare decisions, especially when it comes to the efficacy and safety of medical procedures. Clinical trials assist physicians and policymakers in identifying the most effective and suitable therapies for specific patient populations by methodically comparing interventions to placebo or standard of care. In addition, clinical trials aid in the creation of treatment algorithms, clinical practice guidelines, and regulatory choices, guaranteeing that medical actions are supported by the most significant available data.

A clinical trial consists of several major stages, each of which is intended to address a particular research issue or set of goals. In the first stage, referred to as phase 1, a small sample of healthy volunteers or patients with the target condition are used to examine the safety and also tolerability of a novel medication. Phase 2 trials concentrate on assessing the treatment's initial efficacy and ideal dosage in a larger patient population. Phase 3 trials are more extensive, multicenter studies designed to evaluate a treatment to placebo or standard of care while verifying the safety and effectiveness of the medication across a range of patient categories. Phase 4 trials, which are often referred to as post-marketing surveillance studies, are carried out subsequent to the treatment's approval for usage with the objective of overseeing its long-term safety and efficacy in authentic clinical environments.

The design, conduct, and also oversight of clinical trials are significantly influenced by ethical considerations, which guarantee the safety of study participants and the validity and reliability of research findings. Three fundamental ethical precepts that guide clinical trial research are beneficence, justice, and respect for human dignity. Respect for people demands that people be given the freedom to decide whether or not to participate in research and that their rights to privacy, dignity, and autonomy are upheld. In order for research to be considered beneficent, study subjects must be shielded from harm, and the possible advantages must exceed the hazards. In order to do so, all study participants must share equally in the advantages and burdens associated with it, irrespective of their socioeconomic background or other variables.

Clinical trials have numerous advantages, but they also have a number of drawbacks that may affect their validity, generalizability, and suitability for use in actual clinical settings. Finding and keeping volunteers is a problem, especially when it comes to marginalized or underprivileged groups that can be reluctant to take part in studies. Furthermore, bias, confounding, and other methodological flaws in clinical trials may alter how study results are interpreted. In addition, clinical trials can be costly, time-consuming, and resource-intensive, requiring significant commitments of capital, knowledge, and time to carry out effectively. Lastly, the generalizability and application of clinical trials to a variety of patient groups and healthcare contexts may be limited if they do not accurately represent the diversity of patient populations or real-world clinical settings.

Clinical trial research has a bright future ahead of it, one that will undoubtedly advance healthcare and enhance patient outcomes. Technological advancements like wearables, mobile health apps, and electronic health records allow researchers to run virtual or remote clinical trials, monitor patient results in real-time, and collect data more correctly and efficiently. Furthermore, the effectiveness, adaptability, and relevance of clinical trial research are being enhanced by cutting-edge trial designs like pragmatic, adaptive, and platform trials.

Furthermore, initiatives like patient advocacy, community involvement, and cultural competence training that aim to broaden diversity and inclusivity in clinical trial participation are improving the representativeness and generalizability of research results. Clinical trial research can continue to be a significant contributor to the advancement of medical knowledge, the guidance of clinical practice, and the enhancement of patient care in the years to come by overcoming these obstacles and seizing these opportunities.

To sum up, clinical trials are critical to the advancement of evidence-based medicine in the healthcare industry and the enhancement of patient outcomes. Clinical trials offer essential insights into the most efficient methods for illness prevention, diagnosis, and treatment by methodically assessing the safety, efficacy, and effectiveness of medical therapies and interventions. Clinical trial research has its share of difficulties and restrictions, but further attempts to diversify trial participants, advance trial techniques, and use technology have enormous potential to advance medicine and better patient care in the future. If we continue to build on the successes and insights from clinical trial research, we can ensure that evidence-based practice remains at the forefront of healthcare innovation and delivery.

Herbal Antivirals in Epidemics and Pandemics

Finding efficient therapies and preventative measures is crucial to halting the spread and damaging effects of viral infections during epidemics and pandemics. Although there are many pharmaceutical interventions available in modern medicine, there is growing interest in investigating the potential of herbal antivirals as alternative or complementary therapies. Infectious disorders have traditionally been treated with herbal therapy, and new studies are starting to reveal the antiviral qualities of many therapeutic plants. In this section, we shall examine the role of herbal antivirals in epidemics and pandemics, as well as their modes of action, efficacy evidence, safety concerns, and prospects and obstacles in their application.

Herbal antivirals work in multiple ways, such as by

directly preventing the spread of viruses, influencing the immune system, and bolstering the defenses of the host. Bioactive substances that have antiviral qualities are found in many medicinal plants and include flavonoids, alkaloids, terpenoids, and polyphenols. These substances have been demonstrated to obstruct viral entrance, replication, and assembly. For instance, it has been established that substances present in licorice root (Glycyrrhiza glabra) suppress the reproduction of herpes simplex virus (HSV) and respiratory syncytial virus (RSV) and that extracts from elderberries (Sambucus nigra) exhibit antiviral properties against influenza viruses. Furthermore, it has been discovered that herbal remedies, including Andrographis paniculata, Echinacea purpurea, and Astragalus membranaceus, modify the immune response, strengthening the body's defense against viral infections.

While there is still a lack of evidence to support the effectiveness of herbal antivirals in epidemics and pandemics, a few research have shown encouraging findings. During the H1N1 influenza pandemic, for instance, a randomized controlled trial revealed that an elderberry extract, when compared to a placebo, decreased the length and intensity of symptoms. In a similar vein, Andrographis paniculata was shown to considerably lessen upper respiratory tract infection symptoms when compared to a placebo in a meta-analysis of clinical trials. Although these findings are promising, more investigation is required to validate the effectiveness of herbal antivirals in various viral infections and patient cohorts.

When using herbal antivirals, safety must always come first, especially in times of epidemics and pandemics when a considerable population may be exposed to these medications. Herbal remedies can have adverse effects and interact with other pharmaceuticals despite the fact that they are frequently thought of as natural and safe.

Furthermore, there can be significant variations in the quality and purity of herbal products, raising questions regarding adulteration, contamination, and mislabeling.

The safety and effectiveness of herbal antivirals must be guaranteed by regulatory oversight and quality control procedures, which differ significantly between nations and areas. Patients should be informed about the possible hazards and advantages of herbal antivirals, and healthcare professionals should be cognizant of these factors when recommending them to patients.

In the context of epidemics and pandemics, the use of herbal antivirals presents both opportunities and obstacles, notwithstanding their potential benefits. One issue that can make it challenging to evaluate the safety and also the efficacy of herbal medications is the need for standardized formulations and dosage guidelines.

Furthermore, the infrastructure and funding for research on herbal medicines need to be improved, which leaves gaps in our knowledge of their safety, effectiveness, and mechanisms of action. Yet, academics, medical professionals, and legislators are becoming more aware of the potential of herbal antivirals, and this has resulted in a rise in funding for this field of study and development.

In summary, herbal antivirals may be extremely helpful in the management and avoidance of viral infections during pandemics and epidemics. They are appealing choices to take into consideration because of their variety of modes of action, efficacy proof, and affordability. However, while using them, care must be taken, keeping in mind quality control procedures, safety concerns, and the need for more research. Herbal antivirals have the potential to provide novel approaches for managing viral infections and enhancing public health during pandemics and epidemics by utilizing the natural defense mechanisms found in the environment.

CHAPTER VII

Safety and Regulation of Herbal Antivirals

Navigating Safety Concerns and Adverse Effects

Given their potential to significantly affect patient outcomes and treatment outcomes, safety concerns and adverse effects are important factors to take into account in the healthcare industry. All interventions, whether they be medical equipment, pharmaceuticals, surgery, or complementary and alternative therapies, contain some level of risk. In order to protect patients, healthcare providers must appropriately manage these risks. The numerous safety issues and negative consequences that arise in the healthcare industry, the methods and tactics used to manage and reduce these risks, and the significance of patient-centered care in enhancing safety and minimizing harm will all be covered in this section.

Medication safety is one of the main issues with safety in healthcare since pharmaceuticals are essential to medical care but also carry a risk of adverse drug reactions, prescription errors, and drug interactions. Adverse medication reactions are a primary global source of morbidity and mortality. They can vary from moderate side effects to life-threatening occurrences. In addition to warning patients about possible risks, healthcare providers need to be on the lookout for adverse drug reactions and put medication error prevention measures in place, like computerized physician order entry systems, barcode medication administration, and medication reconciliation procedures. Pharmacovigilance programs, drug safety committees, and interdisciplinary collaboration among healthcare providers are further initiatives to enhance pharmaceutical safety.

Because medical gadgets can malfunction, break down, or injure someone if not utilized correctly, they also raise safety concerns. Medical devices are essential for patient diagnosis, treatment, and follow-up. They range from implanted devices like pacemakers and joint replacements to diagnostic tools like MRI scanners and X-ray machines. If not made, maintained, or constructed correctly, they can potentially present hazards of infections, injuries, or adverse reactions. Medical device maintenance and operation must also be taught to healthcare professionals, and they must be ready to act quickly in the event of a device-related adverse event.

Surgical operations are inherently risky, and even when best practices and recommendations are followed, complications, including infections, bleeding, and organ damage, can still happen. By encouraging uniform practices, teamwork, and preoperative safety checks, surgical safety initiatives—like the World Health Organization's Surgical Safety Checklist—seek to lower the risk of surgical complications. Surgical safety and results have also improved as a result of developments in perioperative care, anesthetic procedures, and surgical techniques. Surgeons, anesthesiologists, nurses, and also other medical personnel must collaborate to identify and manage any risks and guarantee patient safety during the perioperative phase in order to achieve surgical safety.

Recently, supplementary and alternative therapies like herbal therapy, acupuncture, chiropractic adjustments, and mind-body approaches have become more and more popular. However, because these therapies are not regulated, standardized, or supported by scientific research, there are safety issues associated with them. A number of complementary and also alternative medicines can be risky when taken improperly, or they may interact with conventional treatments or cause delays in seeking evidence-based care. Healthcare professionals must converse candidly and openly with patients on the usage of these therapies, as well as their possible advantages and disadvantages. Through the processes of licensing, certification, and accreditation, professional associations and regulatory bodies also contribute to the safety and caliber of complementary and alternative therapies.

Since patient-centered care emphasizes the value of respecting patients' autonomy, interests, and choices, it is crucial for enhancing safety and minimizing harm in the healthcare system. In order to provide patients with patient-centered care, healthcare providers must actively involve patients in their decision-making process, pay attention to their needs and preferences, and offer them the information and support they need to make wise decisions. Critical elements of patient-centered care that enhance safety and lower the chance of unfavorable outcomes include shared decision-making, informed consent, and open communication between patients and healthcare professionals. Furthermore, peer networks, support groups, and patient advocacy organizations can provide patients with the tools they need to actively participate in their own safety and speak up for their needs and preferences in medical settings.

In summary, while harmful consequences and safety issues are unavoidable in the healthcare industry, they can be controlled and lessened with the use of practical tactics. Critical areas of focus for improving patient safety and minimizing injury include medication safety, medical device safety, surgical safety, and safety in complementary and alternative therapies. With its focus on open communication, informed consent, and shared decision-making, patient-centered care is essential for fostering safety and guaranteeing that patients receive high-quality, safe, and efficient treatment. Healthcare professionals can effectively manage safety issues and side effects while providing optimal treatment for their patients by placing a high priority on patient safety and employing evidence-based practices.

Regulatory Frameworks for Herbal Products

Traditional medical systems have been using herbal products to cure and promote health for millennia. But as herbal medicines become more and more popular in today's world, questions have been raised concerning their efficacy, safety, and quality. Many nations have created regulatory frameworks to control the production, promotion, and retailing of herbal products in order to allay these worries. The regulatory frameworks for herbal goods will be discussed in this section, along with their goals, elements, difficulties, and areas for development.

Public health protection, product safety and efficacy, and consumer confidence are the main goals of regulatory regimes for herbal goods. Regulatory bodies are in charge of regulating herbal goods, which includes establishing guidelines for their efficacy, safety, and quality, inspecting and auditing manufacturing facilities, and making sure that regulations are followed. Product registration and licensing, good manufacturing practices (GMP), labeling and packaging specifications, post-market surveillance, and pharmacovigilance are just a few of the elements that regulatory frameworks usually include.

Regulatory frameworks for herbal goods must include product registration and licensing as essential elements since they guarantee that only high-quality, safe, and effective products are permitted for sale. Manufacturers must provide regulatory bodies with thorough paperwork, including information on production procedures, safety, effectiveness, and quality control. The documentation must be reviewed and approved. Product licenses or marketing authorizations are given to products that satisfy regulatory standards, enabling them to be sold to end users. Regulatory bodies may also mandate that producers carry out clinical studies or submit documentation of customary applications in order to substantiate the security and effectiveness of their goods.

Throughout the manufacturing process, rules and guidelines known as good manufacturing practices (GMP) guarantee the quality and uniformity of herbal products. The sourcing of raw materials, product formulation, manufacturing procedures, quality control, packaging, labeling, and storage are all covered by GMP regulations. In order to guarantee that herbal products are produced in a way that reduces the possibility of contamination, adulteration, and variation in potency and composition, adherence to GMP standards is necessary. Regulatory bodies carry out audits and inspections of production sites to confirm adherence to GMP specifications. If manufacturers do not satisfy these requirements, they may face enforcement proceedings.

Regulatory frameworks for herbal goods also include standards for labeling and packaging, which are crucial since they give customers vital information about the product, such as its contents, dose guidelines, indications, contraindications, and precautions. Requirements for labeling may also include directions for safe use, interactions with other medications, and warnings regarding possible adverse effects. Packaging specifications guarantee that herbal goods are stored and transported in containers that guard against contamination, deterioration, and tampering. Regulatory bodies impose adherence to labeling and packaging specifications in order to guarantee that customers can obtain accurate and trustworthy information on herbal goods.

Essential elements of regulatory frameworks for herbal products are post-market monitoring and pharmacovigilance, which enable regulatory bodies to keep an eye on the effectiveness and safety of goods after they are put on the market, as well as to recognize and address adverse occurrences and safety issues. Data on adverse events, problems with product quality, and other safety concerns that are reported by manufacturers, customers, and healthcare providers are gathered and analyzed as part of post-market monitoring. Clinical trials, risk assessments, and epidemiological studies are all part of pharmacovigilance, which assesses the safety and effectiveness of products and provides information for regulatory decision-making. Regulatory bodies utilize this data to implement suitable regulatory measures, such as product recalls, label alerts, or suspensions of marketing, with the aim of safeguarding public health.

Although regulatory frameworks for herbal products are essential, there are a number of obstacles they must overcome and areas where they may be strengthened. One issue is the need for uniformity and harmonization in regulatory standards among various nations and areas, which can obstruct trade and make it more difficult for customers to obtain herbal products. Furthermore, regulatory bodies may need to gain the necessary tools, knowledge, or experience to properly supervise the control of herbal goods, especially in low- and middle-income nations. In addition, authorities need help in keeping up with advancements and guaranteeing the efficacy and safety of products due to the industry's explosive expansion in the herbal products sector and the introduction of novel products and ingredients.

Nonetheless, there exist prospects for enhancing the regulatory frameworks pertaining to herbal products. These opportunities include endeavors to normalize and uniformize regulatory obligations among nations and areas, augment cooperation and exchange of data among regulatory bodies, and fortify post-market surveillance and pharmacovigilance protocols. Furthermore, authorities can confirm the legitimacy, potency, and purity of herbal items as well as identify adulteration and contamination with the use of technological developments in analytical approaches, quality control procedures, and authentication technologies. Additionally, involving stakeholders in the regulation process may guarantee that frameworks are open, inclusive, and sensitive to the needs and worries of all parties involved. These stakeholders include researchers, manufacturers, healthcare practitioners, and consumers.

To sum up, regulatory frameworks are essential for guaranteeing the quality, safety, and effectiveness of herbal products as well as for safeguarding the general public's health. Regulatory bodies assist in guaranteeing that customers have access to safe, efficient, and superior herbal goods by setting rules and guidelines for product registration and licensing, good manufacturing practices, labeling and packaging requirements, and post-market surveillance. Harmonization, consistency, and capacity are issues that regulatory frameworks must deal with, but cooperation, creativity, and stakeholder involvement can help them get better. Regulatory bodies can continue to carry out their responsibility of protecting public health and fostering consumer confidence in herbal products by tackling these issues and making use of these opportunities.

Quality Control and Standardization Measures

Pharmaceutical medications, medical gadgets, and herbal treatments are just a few examples of healthcare items whose manufacturing processes require quality control and standardization. These steps are intended to guarantee that goods are consistent in their composition, potency, and performance and that they adhere to accepted standards of safety, efficacy, and quality. The significance of quality control and standardization in healthcare products, the primary methods and strategies employed to accomplish these goals, and the opportunities and difficulties associated with putting these policies into practice will all be covered in this article.

The term "quality control" refers to a variety of procedures and actions used to keep an eye on and preserve the standard of medical supplies during production. Testing of raw materials, products in production, final products, environmental monitoring, and quality assurance are a few examples of these tasks. To ensure that products fulfill legal criteria and are safe and also effective for their intended purpose, quality control procedures assist in discovering and addressing deviations from set specifications, such as impurities, contaminants, or changes in potency. To further protect public health and reduce liability, quality control assists producers in identifying and reducing the likelihood of product faults, recalls, and unfavorable events.

To guarantee uniformity and consistency in the composition, potency, and performance of healthcare goods, standards, guidelines, and procedures are established and put into practice through the process of standardization. Standardization measures encompass several aspects, such as the creation of uniform formulas, production operations, analytical techniques, and quality control protocols. Manufacturers may guarantee that products are constant in their quality and performance, regardless of when and where they are produced, by standardizing crucial parts of the production process, such as the sourcing of raw materials, product formulation, and testing procedures. Standardization makes it easier to compare items and makes it possible to evaluate safety, effectiveness, and quality more precisely.

Analytical testing, which uses tools and procedures for analysis to determine the identification, purity, potency, and quality of medical items, is one of the main methods used in quality control and standardization. Among the techniques used in analytical testing are spectroscopy, mass spectrometry, chromatography, microbiological assays, and biological assays. In order to make sure that healthcare items adhere to set standards and legal criteria, manufacturers can use these techniques to identify and measure the active substances, contaminants, impurities, and degradation products in those products. Analytical testing also assists in locating and resolving deviations from standard operating procedures that could impact the quality of the product, such as differences in production processes or equipment performance.

Validation is a crucial tool in quality control and standardization processes. It entails proving that manufacturing processes, analytical techniques, and quality control protocols can reliably produce goods that adhere to prescribed specifications and legal requirements. Among other things, validation activities could involve equipment qualification, cleaning validation, process validation, and method validation. Manufacturers may guarantee that their goods are high-quality, safe, and compliant with regulations by verifying essential components of the manufacturing process. Furthermore, validation contributes to the prevention of adverse events, recalls, and product defects by identifying and mitigating risks and safeguarding patient safety as well as public health.

A number of factors, such as the complexity of manufacturing processes, the variability of raw materials, the ever-changing nature of regulatory requirements, and the lack of resources and expertise, can make the implementation of effective quality control and standardization measures difficult, despite their importance. Furthermore, outsourcing manufacturing operations and globalizing supply chains may present new difficulties for collaboration, communication, and monitoring among various stakeholders. Still, there are ways to improve quality control and standardization. Technological developments like automation, robots, and artificial intelligence can improve the processes of quality control and standardization by making them more reliable, accurate, and efficient.

To sum up, consistency and safety in healthcare items are ensured by quality control and standardization procedures. Manufacturers may make sure that their goods fulfill safety, efficacy, and quality standards by putting strict quality control methods in place, such as analytical testing, validation, and quality assurance.

Furthermore, standardization efforts contribute to maintaining consistency and uniformity in the potency, composition, and performance of medical supplies, which improves patient safety and makes product comparison easier. Although putting in place efficient quality control and standardization procedures can be difficult, there are ways to make things better thanks to technological developments, teamwork, and creativity. Manufacturers may continue to supply high-quality, safe, and adequate healthcare goods that satisfy the demands of healthcare professionals and patients by placing a strong priority on quality control and standardization.

CHAPTER VIII

Herbal Antivirals: Future Perspectives

Emerging Trends in Herbal Antiviral Research

The pressing need for efficient treatments for viral infections has led to a rise in interest in research on herbal antivirals in recent years. With its long history and wide range of bioactive chemicals, herbal medicine offers a viable path for the development of new antiviral drugs. Scholars are increasingly drawing inspiration from traditional medicinal plants and indigenous healing methods in an effort to uncover the therapeutic potential concealed within the abundance of nature. This paper investigates the new directions in plant extract antiviral research, such as the identification of novel bioactive components, the investigation of plant extract synergistic effects, and the creation of creative delivery systems.

The identification of new bioactive substances with strong antiviral effects is one of the most critical developments in herbal antiviral research. Herbal remedies, highly valued for their curative qualities in numerous societies across the globe, are demonstrating an abundant supply of bioactive substances capable of regulating immunological reactions, reducing the intensity of viral infections, and inhibiting viral growth.

Thanks to developments in phytochemistry and pharmacology, high-throughput screening methods have made it possible for researchers to extract and discover bioactive substances from medicinal plants that have exceptional antiviral activity. These substances, which include coronaviruses, herpes simplex, flavonoids, alkaloids, terpenoids, and polyphenols, have broad-spectrum activity against a variety of viruses, including influenza, HIV, and herpes simplex.

Examining the potential synergistic effects of plant extracts and traditional antiviral medications is another new direction in herbal antiviral research. Although traditional antiviral medications have been helpful in treating viral infections, the advent of drug-resistant viruses and unfavorable side effects frequently restrict their effectiveness. Herbal extracts present a potential remedy for many issues because of their intricate combinations of bioactive components. Research has indicated that the co-administration of herbal extracts with traditional antiviral medications can augment their effectiveness, mitigate the likelihood of drug resistance, and boost patient outcomes. For instance, it has been discovered that licorice root extract and acyclovir work together to synergistically limit the multiplication of the herpes simplex virus, improving treatment results.

Apart from investigating new bioactive substances and their combined effects, scientists are also concentrating on creating inventive delivery methods for herbal antiviral treatments. There may be drawbacks to using traditional techniques of preparing herbs, such as decoctions, infusions, and tinctures, in terms of patient compliance, stability, and bioavailability. Nanoparticles, liposomes, microspheres, and nanoemulsions are examples of novel delivery methods that have advantages in terms of targeted distribution, controlled release, and improved absorption of bioactive substances. With the use of these delivery methods, herbal antivirals' pharmacokinetics and pharmacodynamics can be enhanced, improving treatment success and minimizing side effects.

Moreover, knowledge exchange and interdisciplinary cooperation are essential forces behind progress in the field of herbal antiviral research. Scholars from several disciplines, including virology, immunology, pharmacology, phytochemistry, and nanotechnology, are collaborating to address the intricate problems associated with viral infections. Research discoveries are being translated into clinical applications more quickly because of cooperation between government, business, and academic institutions. This will guarantee that promising herbal antivirals are brought to market and help patients all over the world.

Research on herbal antivirals has advanced, but there are still a number of obstacles to overcome. The requirement for established techniques to assess the security, effectiveness, and caliber of herbal antiviral treatments is one difficulty. For herbal products, regulatory bodies want proof of safety, effectiveness, and quality control. This proof might take the form of data from preclinical and clinical research, analytical test findings, and manufacturing process documentation. For research results and regulatory decision-making to be consistent and reliable, standardized procedures for assessing herbal antivirals are crucial.

The variation in the makeup and strength of herbal medicines brought about by elements such as plant genetics, cultivation circumstances, harvesting techniques, and processing procedures presents another difficulty. To ensure uniformity in their potency, composition, and performance—and to enable more precise evaluations of their safety, efficacy, and quality— herbal products must be standardized. However, the diversity of plant matrices and the existence of several bioactive chemicals with antagonistic or synergistic effects might make standardization challenging to achieve.

To sum up, research on herbal antivirals is an exciting and quickly developing topic that has great promise to alleviate the global burden of viral infections. There is new hope in the fight against viral illnesses thanks to emerging developments in herbal antiviral research, such as the identification of novel bioactive components, the investigation of synergistic effects with conventional antiviral medications, and the creation of creative delivery systems. Herbal antiviral research can progress and help provide safe, efficient, and readily available therapies for viral infections by tackling issues including uniformity, variability, and the requirement for more thorough clinical study.

The Promise of Personalized Herbal Medicine

Personalized medicine is a new and innovative field in healthcare that aims to improve treatment outcomes by customizing medical therapies to the specific needs of each patient. Herbal medicine is a field where tailored techniques have gained recognition despite personalized medicine being generally connected with genetic therapies and pharmaceutical medications. Phytopersonalization, another name for personalized herbal therapy, is a prospective paradigm change in healthcare that utilizes a variety of plant-based medicines to meet each patient's unique needs. This section will examine the potential of customized herbal therapy, outlining its foundational ideas, clinical uses, obstacles, and prospects for growth.

The understanding that every person is biochemically unique, with a unique genetic composition, physiological traits, exposure to the environment, and lifestyle choices that affect health and disease, is the foundation of personalized herbal therapy. Personalized herbal medicine considers these individual variations in order to determine which herbal therapies are best for each patient, taking into consideration their unique health problems, preferences, and treatment reactions. With this individualized approach, medical professionals can customize herbal remedies to target the underlying causes of illness, maximize therapeutic benefits, reduce side effects, and improve patient compliance and satisfaction.

The idea of constitutional medicine, which distinguishes between several constitutional kinds or body constitutions based on conventional medical systems like Traditional Chinese Medicine (TCM), Ayurveda, and Unani medicine, is one of the fundamental tenets of customized herbal treatment. These systems divide people into different constitutional types according to their physical attributes, temperament, and imbalance patterns. Healthcare professionals can choose herbal medicines that are especially suited to each patient's unique constitution and health demands by determining their constitutional type. This helps to maximize therapeutic advantages and reduce the possibility of unfavorable reactions.

Personalized herbal medicine integrates the ideas of precision medicine, which uses genomic data, diagnostic tests, and biomarkers to customize treatment plans for each patient, in addition to constitutional medicine. Technological developments like metabolomics, microbiome analysis, and genetic sequencing are making it possible for scientists to find biomarkers that can predict a person's reaction to herbal therapy and direct individualized treatment plans. The metabolism and effectiveness of herbal treatments may be influenced by genetic variations in drug-metabolizing enzymes, such as cytochrome P450 enzymes. This information enables medical professionals to modify dosages and treatment plans accordingly.

Numerous medical ailments, including chronic illnesses, autoimmune diseases, metabolic abnormalities, and mental health issues, are treated clinically with individualized herbal medication. Herbs with anti-inflammatory qualities for patients with inflammatory bowel disease, adaptogenic properties for patients with disorders related to stress, or hepatoprotective qualities for patients with liver disease are a few examples of the kinds of herbs that may be included in customized herbal protocols. Personalized herbal therapy provides the possibility of more accurate and successful treatments that enhance patient outcomes and quality of life by adjusting herbal therapies to target the unique underlying causes and processes of disease in each individual patient.

Although personalized herbal medicine has a lot of potential, many challenges need to be solved before it can be applied extensively in clinical settings. The absence of defined methods and protocols for customized herbal prescriptions—which might differ significantly based on the preferences, education, and experience of each practitioner—is one issue. Furthermore, additional study is required to confirm the effectiveness, safety, and affordability of customized herbal medicine methods using carefully planned clinical trials and observational studies. Regulatory concerns about labeling, standardization, and quality control of herbal products make it challenging to incorporate customized herbal therapy into traditional healthcare systems.

The use of customized herbal medicine is also fraught with ethical issues and cultural sensitivities, especially when combined with conventional medical procedures and indigenous knowledge systems. The development and application of customized herbal medicine approaches must be guided by fundamental concepts such as respect for cultural variety, traditional wisdom, and community engagement. Working together and having conversations with contemporary medical professionals and traditional healers can help close the gap between various healing traditions and promote mutual trust, respect, and understanding.

Notwithstanding these obstacles, customized herbal therapy presents a wealth of chances for progress and creativity in the medical field. By encouraging preventive care, patient empowerment, and holistic approaches to health and wellness, integrating customized herbal medicine into traditional healthcare systems can increase treatment options, enhance patient outcomes, and lower healthcare costs. Customized herbal medicine has the potential to transform healthcare and also usher in a new era of individualized, patient-centered treatment that prioritizes individual health requirements and preferences by embracing the concepts of personalized medicine and harnessing the restorative power of nature.

Creating a Bridge Between Scientific Innovation and Conventional Knowledge

There is much to be discovered and explored in a variety of sectors, including technology, agriculture, medicine, and ecology, at the nexus of traditional knowledge and scientific innovation. A wealth of information and insight into the natural world and its workings can be gained from traditional knowledge, which has been amassed over generations via observation, experimentation, and cultural traditions. In the meantime, scientific innovation, propelled by developments in technology, research techniques, and multidisciplinary cooperation, aims to deepen our comprehension of the world and provide fresh approaches to challenging problems. This section will discuss the significance of bridging the gap between scientific innovation and traditional knowledge, the opportunities and problems that come with this attempt, and the possibility of collaboration and synergy between the two methods.

Herbal medicine, farming methods, environmental preservation, and spiritual beliefs are just a few of the fields covered by traditional knowledge, which is frequently transmitted orally, culturally, and through indigenous healing systems. The close interaction that exists between people and their surroundings is reflected in this knowledge, which is firmly anchored in regional ecosystems, cultural values, and interpersonal relationships. The transmission of knowledge from one generation to the next is facilitated by traditional healers, elders, and knowledge holders. This ensures the continuity and applicability of the knowledge in modern settings. Traditional knowledge can adapt to changing social, environmental, and economic conditions because it is dynamic and adaptive.

On the other hand, scientific innovation produces new knowledge and creative solutions to complex issues through methodical investigation, empirical data, and strict procedures. Our ability to view, analyze, and influence the natural environment at different scales, from the molecular to the global, has been revolutionized by technological advancements like genetics, nanotechnology, and artificial intelligence. The integration of insights from varied domains and methodologies to handle complex difficulties is made possible by interdisciplinary collaboration and open exchange of ideas, which are fundamental elements that propel scientific innovation.

Traditional knowledge and scientific innovation have different methods and approaches. Still, they are united by a shared commitment to bettering human well-being, understanding the natural world, and advancing sustainable development. We may make use of the complementing qualities of both methods and open up new avenues for advancement by bridging the gap between conventional knowledge and scientific innovation. For instance, scientific studies on conservation biology, climate change adaptation, and ecosystem restoration can benefit from the inclusion of traditional ecological knowledge, which includes indigenous peoples' understanding of ecosystems, biodiversity, and sustainable resource management.

Personalized treatment modalities, holistic approaches to health and wellness, and the medicinal qualities of medicinal plants are all provided by traditional medicine systems, including Traditional Chinese Medicine (TCM), Ayurveda, and Indigenous healing traditions. The amalgamation of conventional medicine with contemporary biomedical research and clinical practice has the potential to augment patient care, elevate therapy results, and broaden treatment alternatives for intricate and persistent ailments. Research on the pharmacological characteristics of medicinal plants, for instance, that are employed in traditional medical systems, has produced new bioactive chemicals that may find value in drug development and natural product-based treatments.

However, there are obstacles to overcome in order to bridge the gap between conventional wisdom and scientific innovation effectively. Respecting, comprehending, and appreciating the worth of indigenous intellectual property rights and also traditional knowledge systems is one difficulty. Indigenous communities frequently experience marginalization, exploitation, and cultural appropriation of their traditional knowledge by governments, companies, and scholars, among other external entities. Ensuring fair partnerships, mutual benefit, and informed consent in joint research and innovation endeavors requires respecting indigenous sovereignty, self-determination, and cultural customs.

Furthermore, obstacles to efficient communication and cooperation can include linguistic difficulties, cultural disparities, and variations in the epistemology of traditional knowledge and scientific paradigms. Oral traditions, metaphors, and symbols are common ways that traditional knowledge is passed down; these can be difficult to transfer into scientific language or procedures. Furthermore, traditional knowledge systems could give weight to viewpoints that diverge from Western science, including alternative values, worldviews, and methods of knowing. It will take humility, perseverance, and open-mindedness on the part of researchers, policymakers, and practitioners working on collaborative initiatives to bridge these cultural and epistemological gaps.

In order to guarantee that cooperative research and innovation initiatives fulfill the values of justice, fairness, and respect for human rights, ethical issues, including informed consent, community involvement, and intellectual property rights, must also be appropriately taken into account. The right to manage and profit from traditional knowledge should belong to indigenous peoples and local communities. This includes the authority to determine its appropriate uses, distribution, and preservation. Equitable involvement, joint knowledge production, and benefit exchange between all parties involved should be given top priority in collaborative research and innovation collaborations.

Conclusively, establishing a bridge between conventional knowledge and scientific innovation has immense prospects for exploration, cooperation, and advancement across diverse domains. We may create more comprehensive, contextually relevant, and long-lasting answers to the complex problems that confront both humanity and the environment by fusing ideas from traditional knowledge systems with scientific research and innovation. To be successful, this project calls for equitable relationships, ethical thinking, mutual respect, and an appreciation of the importance of traditional knowledge. We can create a more harmonic and inclusive approach to knowledge generation, problem-solving, and sustainable development by integrating the complementary qualities of scientific innovation and traditional wisdom.

CHAPTER IX

Ethnobotanical Insights into Herbal Antivirals

Cultural Perspectives on Herbal Medicine

For millennia, herbal medicine has been an essential component of human civilization, permeating the customs, ideologies, and lifestyles of several global communities. Cultural viewpoints on herbal medicine provide an intriguing glimpse into the intricate interactions between historical, social, ecological, and spiritual elements that influence how we perceive and utilize therapeutic herbs. The rich tapestry of human experience and the enduring bond between humans and the natural world is reflected in the diversity of cultural viewpoints on herbal therapy. These perspectives range from ancient healing traditions passed down through generations to contemporary practices influenced by globalization and modernization. We will examine the many facets of herbal medicine from cultural perspectives in this thorough investigation, looking at its historical origins, cultural importance, therapeutic applications, and current applicability in many cultural contexts across the globe.

Herbal medicine has a long history that extends back to the earliest known civilizations in Mesopotamia, Egypt, China, and the Indus Valley. In fact, its history predates human civilization itself. Herbal medicine has long been an integral part of the healing traditions of many different civilizations, from the Sumerians' use of medicinal herbs in ancient Mesopotamia to the herbal pharmacopeias of ancient Egypt and China. Globally, indigenous peoples have created intricate systems of herbal medicine based on cultural practices, oral traditions, and empirical observation that have been passed down through the years. Native American tribes in the Americas, such as the Maya, Aztecs, and Inca, utilized medicinal plants for daily health care as well as healing rites and spiritual ceremonies. Comparably, for thousands of years, indigenous healing practices in Africa, Australia, and the Pacific Islands, Traditional Chinese Medicine (TCM) in China, and Ayurveda in India have preserved and transmitted herbal knowledge while adjusting to shifting social, cultural, and environmental circumstances.

In many communities, herbal medicine is deeply ingrained in culture, acting as a pillar of social cohesiveness, spirituality, and cultural identity in addition to providing treatment. Medicinal plants are frequently seen as holy gifts from the ground, representing the interdependence of all living things and the knowledge of the ancestors. Shamans, medicine women, and traditional healers all have essential roles to play in maintaining community health, preserving herbal knowledge, and serving as intermediaries between the spirit and human realms. Deeply ingrained in cultural customs, herbal medicine rituals, ceremonies, and practices commemorate significant life events, seasonal shifts, and rites of passage. The use of medicinal plants is entwined with spiritual beliefs, cosmological frameworks, and ecological stewardship in many indigenous cultures. This illustrates a holistic approach to health and wellness that considers the mental, emotional, spiritual, and physical facets of human existence.

Cultural viewpoints on herbal medicine cover a broad spectrum of therapeutic modalities, including mental, emotional, and spiritual components of health and wellness, in addition to the physical parts of treatment. According to traditional healing traditions, illness results from disturbances or imbalances in these essential forces, and health is defined as a condition of harmony and balance between the body, mind, and spirit. By targeting the root causes of illness, bolstering the body's natural healing processes, and encouraging holistic well-being, herbal treatments help to re-establish this balance. To treat disease and advance health, traditional healers frequently combine nutritional advice, lifestyle changes, medicinal herbs, and spiritual practices. Cultural ceremonies, rituals, and practices that foster social support, community cohesiveness, and collective healing also incorporate herbal medicine. To bring harmony and balance back to individuals and communities, healing ceremonies in many indigenous cultures, for instance, may incorporate the use of medicinal plants, chanting, drumming, and dancing.

Herbal medicine still plays a significant role in many cultures throughout the world, providing millions of people with their primary source of healthcare even in the face of contemporary medical advancements. Herbal medicine continues to be an essential source of reasonably priced, easily accessible, and culturally sensitive treatment in developing nations with limited access to conventional healthcare. As individuals embrace holistic approaches to health, look for alternatives to traditional therapies, and rediscover the healing wisdom of their ancestors, there is a growing interest in herbal therapy, even in industrialized nations. Numerous traditional herbal medicines have been validated by scientific studies on medicinal plants, which have confirmed their therapeutic efficacy and safety through rigorous clinical trials and pharmacological tests. Herbal therapy is becoming more widely acknowledged as a valuable adjunct to traditional medicine, providing distinct therapeutic advantages, fewer adverse effects, and a more comprehensive approach to health and well-being.

Cultural viewpoints on herbal medicine provide a complex lens through which to see the diversity of human cultures, the intricate interrelationships between humans and the natural world, and the adaptability of traditional treatment methods in the face of globalization and technology. We can better understand the wisdom of traditional healing methods, the interdependence of humans and the natural world, and the possibility of cross-cultural dialogue and cooperation in the search for health and healing by accepting cultural viewpoints on herbal medicine. Let us remember the priceless lessons and insights that cultural perspectives on herbal medicine give as we negotiate the difficulties of contemporary healthcare. These perspectives serve as a constant reminder of the enduring power of community, tradition, and nature to promote health and well-being for all.

Indigenous Knowledge Systems and Traditional Practices

Indigenous knowledge systems and traditional practices represent a treasure trove of wisdom accumulated over centuries by indigenous peoples around the world. Rooted in deep connections to land, nature, and community, indigenous knowledge encompasses a holistic understanding of the world, encompassing diverse fields such as medicine, agriculture, ecology, spirituality, and governance. Traditional practices passed down through generations via oral traditions, rituals, ceremonies, and practical experiences are essential for the survival, resilience, and cultural identity of indigenous communities. In this comprehensive exploration, we will delve into the multifaceted world of indigenous knowledge systems and traditional practices, examining their historical roots, cultural significance, ecological relevance, and contemporary challenges and opportunities in the context of sustainable development and cultural preservation.

Indigenous knowledge systems have deep historical roots, dating back thousands of years to the dawn of human civilization. Indigenous peoples have developed sophisticated ways of understanding and interacting with their environments based on intimate relationships with local ecosystems, ancestral teachings, and collective experiences. Traditional knowledge systems encompass a wide range of domains, including medicinal plants, hunting and gathering practices, weather prediction, land stewardship, storytelling, and cultural ceremonies. These knowledge systems are embedded in cultural traditions, cosmological beliefs, and social structures that reflect the unique histories, values, and worldviews of indigenous cultures. For example, indigenous healing practices, such as Traditional Chinese Medicine (TCM), Ayurveda, and Indigenous healing traditions, emphasize the interconnectedness of mind, body, and spirit and the importance of restoring balance and harmony to achieve health and wellness.

Traditional practices are central to the cultural identity, spiritual well-being, and social cohesion of indigenous communities. Rituals, ceremonies, and cultural practices are performed to mark important life events, seasonal transitions, and communal gatherings, reinforcing cultural values, beliefs, and traditions. Traditional knowledge holders, elders, and spiritual leaders play vital roles as custodians of indigenous knowledge, passing down ancestral teachings and wisdom to future generations. Traditional practices are also closely intertwined with land-based activities, such as agriculture, hunting, fishing, and foraging, which sustain indigenous livelihoods and subsistence economies. These practices reflect a deep reverence for nature, biodiversity, and the interconnected web of life, embodying principles of reciprocity, stewardship, and sustainability that are essential for the well-being of both humans and the environment.

Indigenous knowledge systems are intricately linked to local ecosystems and biodiversity, providing valuable insights into ecological processes, resource management, and sustainable living practices. Indigenous peoples have developed sophisticated ways of observing, understanding, and adapting to their environments based on generations of accumulated wisdom and practical experiences. Traditional ecological knowledge encompasses a deep understanding of plant and animal species, habitats, seasonal cycles, and weather patterns, as well as traditional land management practices, such as agroforestry, rotational grazing, and fire management. These practices promote biodiversity conservation, soil fertility, water quality, and resilience to climate change, contributing to the long-term sustainability of ecosystems and also the well-being of indigenous communities. Indigenous knowledge systems emphasize the need to combine traditional ecological knowledge with Western scientific approaches for more equitable and prosperous outcomes, and they offer significant insights into contemporary environmental conservation and resource management activities.

Despite their resilience and adaptability, indigenous knowledge systems and traditional practices face numerous challenges in the modern world, including globalization, environmental degradation, cultural assimilation, and socio-economic marginalization. Rapid urbanization, industrialization, and extractive industries have encroached upon indigenous territories, disrupting traditional ways of life and undermining indigenous peoples' rights to land, resources, and self-determination. Cultural erosion, language loss, and the erosion of traditional knowledge pose further threats to indigenous cultures and identities. Additionally, climate change, deforestation, pollution, and habitat loss are putting pressure on indigenous communities and their traditional livelihoods, exacerbating vulnerabilities and inequalities.

However, there are also opportunities for revitalizing and preserving indigenous knowledge systems and traditional practices in the context of sustainable development and cultural preservation. Indigenous-led initiatives, community-based conservation projects, and partnerships with local and international organizations are helping to empower indigenous communities, strengthen cultural resilience, and promote sustainable livelihoods based on traditional knowledge and practices. Indigenous peoples are increasingly recognized as custodians of biodiversity and guardians of traditional knowledge, with important roles to play in environmental conservation, climate change mitigation, and sustainable development. By respecting indigenous rights, fostering intercultural dialogue, and supporting indigenous-led initiatives, we can harness the wisdom of indigenous knowledge systems and traditional practices to build a more equitable, resilient, and sustainable future for all.

Ethnopharmacological Studies on Antiviral Herbs

Due to the rising incidence of viral infections and the shortcomings of current antiviral treatments, there has been an increase in interest in the potential of traditional herbal remedies as antiviral agents in recent years. The identification and validation of the therapeutic qualities of medicinal plants utilized in traditional treatment systems across the globe depend heavily on ethnopharmacological research. The efficacy, safety, and potential of antiviral herbs for the prevention and also treatment of viral infections are all greatly enhanced by ethnopharmacological research, which documents traditional knowledge, performs pharmacological experiments, and clarifies the underlying mechanisms of action. This section will look at the fundamentals and procedures of ethnopharmacological research on antiviral plants, highlight significant discoveries from studies, and talk about the consequences for traditional medicine, public health, and drug development.

In order to investigate the customary applications of medicinal plants by indigenous peoples and local groups, ethnopharmacology is an interdisciplinary field that incorporates components of ethnobotany, pharmacology, anthropology, and biomedicine. A number of essential steps are usually involved in ethnopharmacological studies on antiviral herbs: phytochemical analysis to identify bioactive compounds, ethnobotanical surveys to record traditional knowledge, pharmacological assays to evaluate antiviral activity, and mechanistic studies to clarify the mechanism of action. In order to guarantee cultural sensitivity, respect for traditional knowledge, and ethical considerations, these studies are frequently carried out in cooperation with indigenous healers, traditional medicine practitioners, and local communities.

For the purpose of recording the customary applications of medicinal plants in various cultures and geographical areas, ethnobotanical surveys are crucial. To gather data on the local flora, medicinal plants, and traditional treatment methods, researchers interview traditional healers, herbalists, and community members. The variety of plant species utilized in traditional medicine, their geographic distribution, and the preparation techniques and dosage forms utilized are all revealed by ethnobotanical surveys. Through the documentation of traditional knowledge, scientists are able to prioritize plants with proven antiviral effects for pharmacological examination and identify prospective candidate plants for additional research.

The process of identifying and characterizing the bioactive substances found in medicinal plants is known as phytochemical analysis. Scholars employ many analytical methodologies, including mass spectrometry, spectroscopy, and chromatography, to separate and recognize phytochemicals that have possible antiviral properties. Alkaloids, flavonoids, terpenoids, phenolics, polysaccharides, and other secondary metabolites with established antiviral activities are a few examples of these bioactive substances. Through the correlation of phytochemical profiles with conventional applications and pharmacological activities, scientists are able to identify the active ingredients accountable for the noted antiviral effects and refine extraction techniques to optimize medicinal performance.

Pharmacological experiments are performed to assess the antiviral efficacy of isolated compounds or extracts from medicinal plants against certain viral infections. Plant extracts are frequently tested for their capacity to prevent viral replication, attachment, entrance, fusion, or other phases of the virus life cycle using in vitro techniques such as cell culture models and enzyme inhibition experiments. Herbal treatments can also be tested in vivo for safety, effectiveness, and pharmacokinetics using animal models in vivo investigations. Pharmacological assays help identify lead compounds for further development as antiviral medicines and provide objective evidence of antiviral action.

The goal of mechanistic research is to clarify the mechanism of action that underlies the antiviral properties of medicinal plants and the bioactive substances they contain. Researchers look into the physiological processes, signaling routes, and molecular targets involved in blocking the spread or reproduction of viruses. Mechanistic studies that observe viral interactions with host cells can use electron microscopy, gene expression analysis, receptor binding assays, and molecular docking simulations. Researchers can enhance drug design, create combination therapies, and find possible pharmacological targets for antiviral intervention by comprehending the molecular processes of action.

Many of the medicinal plants with strong antiviral qualities that have been utilized for generations in traditional medicine have been found through ethnopharmacological research. For instance, extracts from plants with broad-spectrum antiviral activity against respiratory viruses, such as influenza, respiratory syncytial virus (RSV), and coronaviruses, include Andrographis paniculata, Echinacea purpurea, Glycyrrhiza glabra, Sambucus nigra, and Astragalus membranaceus. Bioactive substances found in these plants, including astragalosides, glycyrrhizin, andrographolide, as well as elderberry flavonoids, have been demonstrated to suppress viral replication, alter immunological responses, and strengthen host defenses against viral infections.

The creation of novel antiviral treatments and drug discovery both benefit significantly from ethnopharmacological research. By confirming the traditional uses of medicinal plants and discovering lead compounds with antiviral activity, researchers can expedite the identification of novel pharmaceutical candidates for the prevention as well as treatment of viral infections. Examples of traditional medical systems that offer insightful knowledge on herbal remedies and treatment modalities that can be employed in conjunction with Western medical approaches are Ayurveda, Traditional Chinese Medicine (TCM), and Indigenous healing practices. Modern pharmacology and biomedicine combined with traditional medicine can lead to better treatment outcomes, speed up the process of discovery, and encourage culturally competent healthcare practices that uphold indigenous rights and traditional knowledge.

Research on antiviral herbs through ethnopharmacological studies provides a viable way to investigate nature's pharmacy and find novel remedies for viral illnesses. Researchers can unleash the therapeutic potential of medicinal plants and create potent antiviral medicines that are accessible, affordable, and safe for everyone by fusing traditional wisdom with cutting-edge scientific techniques. In the quest for global health and well-being, ethnopharmacology serves as a link between conventional knowledge systems and biomedical research, encouraging cooperation, respect for one another, and cross-cultural interchange. Ethnopharmacological research gives us hope for utilizing plants' curative properties and securing the future of traditional medicine as we continue to confront the problems of new viral infections and antibiotic resistance.

CHAPTER X

Pharmacokinetics and Pharmacodynamics of Herbal Antivirals

Absorption, Distribution, Metabolism, and Excretion (ADME) of Plant Compounds

In herbal medicine, plant chemicals' absorption, distribution, metabolism, and excretion (ADME) are critical factors in evaluating their safety, effectiveness, and therapeutic potential. Herbal medications are complex mixes of bioactive substances that can interact with different physiological processes in the body, in contrast to synthetic drugs, which are often single chemical entities with well-defined pharmacokinetic characteristics. Optimizing plant chemicals' pharmacological effects, anticipating drug-drug interactions, and guaranteeing their safe and efficient use in clinical practice all depend on an understanding of their ADME characteristics. This section will cover the fundamentals and workings of ADME in relation to herbal medicine, as well as essential variables that affect the pharmacokinetics of plant-based chemicals and their implications for evidence-based medicine, personalized medicine, and drug development.

The process by which plant components are absorbed into the bloodstream following delivery is referred to as absorption. Herbal medications can be injected, breathed, or given topically, although oral intake is the most popular method of delivery. Plant chemicals are primarily absorbed in the gastrointestinal tract, where they pass through the intestinal epithelium and enter the blood. A number of variables, such as a plant compound's chemical makeup, dose form, formulation, and interactions with other medications and food, affect how bioavailable it is. For instance, substances having a high molecular weight or low water solubility may not be well absorbed orally. However, there may be less systemic exposure in those who are highly lipophilic or go through a lot of first-pass metabolism. Furthermore, the pharmacokinetic profile of plant chemicals can be further influenced by interactions with food components, including dietary fibers, lipids, and proteins, which can impact the pace and amount of absorption.

The process via which plant chemicals are dispersed throughout the body following absorption is referred to as distribution. Plant chemicals enter the bloodstream and are subsequently transported by systemic circulation to different tissues and organs. Tissue perfusion, blood-brain barrier penetration, and protein binding are some of the mechanisms that affect the distribution of plant chemicals. Due to their high lipophilicity and ease of passage across cell membranes, a variety of plant chemicals can accumulate in lipid-rich areas such as adipose tissue. Plant chemicals' distribution can also be influenced by protein binding; compounds that are firmly bound to proteins show restricted tissue penetration and slower clearance. Furthermore, plant chemicals may have limited therapeutic effects in both compartments due to restrictions on their access to the central nervous system and fetal circulation, respectively, caused by the blood-brain and placental barriers.

The process by which plant components are biotransformed into metabolites by the body's enzymes is referred to as metabolism. Plant chemicals are mainly metabolized in the liver, while biotransformation events can also occur in the colon, kidney, and lung, among other organs and tissues. Phase I and phase II metabolic reactions, including oxidation, reduction, hydrolysis, conjugation, and methylation, are involved in the metabolism of plant chemicals. These metabolic processes can produce metabolites that are more polar and water-soluble, making it easier for the body to eliminate them through bile or urine. Many components of herbs act as substrates, inducers, or inhibitors of cytochrome P450 (CYP) enzymes, which are essential to the metabolism of plant chemicals. Individual variations in CYP enzyme activity, genetic polymorphisms, and medication interactions affect how plant chemicals are metabolized, resulting in varying pharmacokinetics and therapeutic outcomes.

The removal of plant components and their metabolites from the body is referred to as excretion. Plant chemicals are primarily excreted by the kidneys through urine and the liver through feces. For water-soluble metabolites, renal excretion is the main pathway; however, for lipophilic substances and their metabolites, biliary excretion is more critical. By filtering plant chemicals from the bloodstream into the urine through glomerular filtration, tubular secretion, and tubular reabsorption, the kidney plays a critical role in their disposal. Hepatocytes secrete plant chemicals and their metabolites into bile, which is then excreted from the body through feces. This process is known as biliary excretion. Plant chemicals can have a longer half-life in the body and a different pharmacokinetic profile if they are reabsorbed into the bloodstream through enterohepatic circulation, which is the process by which bile acids and metabolites are taken up from the intestine.

Optimizing plant chemicals' pharmacological effects, anticipating drug-drug interactions, and guaranteeing their safe and efficient use in clinical practice all depend on an understanding of their ADME characteristics. The bioavailability, tissue distribution, metabolic stability, and elimination kinetics of plant chemicals in humans are all greatly aided by pharmacokinetic investigations, which cover absorption, distribution, metabolism, and excretion. To maximize therapeutic efficacy and also reduce side effects, researchers can optimize drug formulations, dosage schedules, and administration methods by clarifying the mechanisms of action and pharmacokinetic features of plant components. Pharmacokinetic studies can also be used to find potential drug interactions, contraindications, and safety issues related to using conventional medications and herbal remedies at the same time. Pharmacokinetic data integration with evidence-based practice can support customized treatment plans, well-informed decision-making, and patient counseling about the safe and efficient use of herbal remedies in clinical settings.

In conclusion, the pharmacokinetic profile and therapeutic benefits of plant components in herbal medicine are greatly influenced by their absorption, distribution, metabolism, and excretion (ADME). Researchers can forecast the pharmacokinetics of plant compounds, enhance their pharmacological qualities, and guarantee the safe and efficient use of these compounds in clinical practice by comprehending the fundamentals and workings of ADME. Pharmacokinetic studies offer essential information about the tissue distribution, bioavailability, metabolic fate, and elimination kinetics of plant chemicals in humans. This information is helpful in informing the creation of new medications, formulations, and evidence-based herbal medicine practices. With the growing popularity of herbal medicine, it will be crucial to incorporate pharmacokinetic data into clinical practice and research to use plant components' therapeutic potential fully and to ensure their safe and efficient application for the betterment of public health and wellbeing.

Pharmacological Mechanisms Underlying Herbal Antiviral Actions

For decades, herbal therapy has been used to treat a wide range of illnesses, including viral infections. The antiviral properties of medicinal plants are attributed to a variety of complex pharmacological mechanisms, many of which involve complex interactions between plant chemicals and viral targets within the host organism. Comprehending these pathways is essential to clarifying the medicinal possibilities of herbal treatments, refining treatment approaches, and creating new antiviral drugs. The pharmacological mechanisms of medicinal plants' antiviral effects, such as host cell protection, immunological modulation, suppression of viral replication, and inhibition of viral entrance, will be discussed in this section. Through the process of deciphering the molecular mechanisms by which herbal substances elicit their antiviral effects, we will be able to leverage nature's pharmacy to fight viral diseases and advance world health.

Viral entrance inhibition is one of the main pharmacological mechanisms by which medicinal herbs exert their antiviral effects. Numerous viruses depend on particular attachment factors or cell surface receptors to enter host cells and start the infection process. By preventing receptor binding, preventing viral fusion with host cell membranes, or impairing viral attachment to target cells, herbal remedies can obstruct viral entrance.

Flavonoids, for instance, are present in plants like licorice (Glycyrrhiza glabra) and green tea (Camellia sinensis), and they have been demonstrated to impede the entry of influenza viruses by preventing the binding of viral hemagglutinin to host cell receptors. In a similar vein, it has been discovered that polysaccharides from plants such as Astragalus membranaceus and Lycium barbarum hinder the herpes simplex virus's (HSV) ability to bind to host cells, hence blocking the virus's entry and subsequent infection.

Herbal antiviral activities also have the essential pharmacological mechanism of suppressing virus replication within infected host cells. Once within the host cell, viruses exploit the machinery of the cell to generate viral proteins, duplicate their genetic information, and put together new viral particles. Various phases of the viral replication cycle, such as protein synthesis, virion assembly, and viral genome replication, can be targeted by herbal remedies. For instance, it has been demonstrated that plant-based polyphenols like curcumin, which is found in turmeric, and resveratrol, which is found in grapes and red wine, prevent the spread of the HIV virus by obstructing reverse transcriptase activity or interfering with viral integrase function. Similar to this, it has been discovered that alkaloids derived from plants such as Hydrastis canadensis and Berberis vulgaris inhibit the hepatitis B virus (HBV) by preventing the development of viral capsids or by reducing the activity of the viral DNA polymerase.

By adjusting the host immune system's reaction to viral infections, herbal medications can also have antiviral effects. Viral pathogens are recognized and eliminated by the immune system, which is responsible for coordinating the antiviral defensive mechanisms through a variety of immune cells and chemicals. Herbal remedies can improve the innate immune system's ability to produce interferons, cytokines, and natural killer cells—all of which aid in preventing the growth and replication of viruses. Herbal remedies can also influence adaptive immune responses, which provide long-term immunity against viral infections. These responses include T cell and B cell activation, antibody formation, and antigen presentation. For instance, polysaccharides from medicinal mushrooms like Lentinula edodes and Ganoderma lucidum have been demonstrated to increase natural killer cell activity and induce the synthesis of interferons, improving antiviral defense against herpes and influenza viruses. Comparably, it has been discovered that flavonoids from plants such as Sambucus nigra and Echinacea purpurea increase phagocytosis and pro-inflammatory cytokine production, therefore facilitating viral clearance and immune activation.

Herbal remedies not only directly combat viral pathogens but also shield host cells from the harm and inflammation caused by viruses, reducing the intensity of viral infections and encouraging tissue regeneration and repair. Infected host cells can experience oxidative stress, inflammation, and apoptosis as a result of viral infections, which can result in tissue damage and malfunction. Herbal remedies that possess cytoprotective, anti-inflammatory, and antioxidant qualities can aid in reducing these pathological processes, maintaining cellular integrity, and enhancing host cell viability.

Phenolic chemicals, for instance, have been demonstrated to scavenge free radicals, suppress inflammatory mediators, and shield host cells from virally-induced oxidative damage. These compounds are present in plants like olive (Olea europaea) and green tea (Camellia sinensis). Similar to this, it has been discovered that terpenoids from plants like Panax ginseng and Ginkgo biloba suppress viral-induced apoptosis and increase cell viability, minimizing tissue damage and enhancing clinical results in viral infections.

The various and complicated interactions between plant chemicals and viral targets within the host organism are the pharmacological mechanisms that underlie the antiviral activities of therapeutic plants. Herbal remedies can have antiviral solid effects and provide promising therapeutic approaches for the prevention and treatment of viral infections by focusing on viral entrance, replication, immunological modulation, and host cell defense. By utilizing nature's pharmacy, scientists can find new antiviral drugs, improve treatment plans, and create creative strategies to fight viral infections. The arsenal of antiviral treatments can be expanded, treatment outcomes can be enhanced, and global health and well-being can be promoted by incorporating herbal medicine into conventional healthcare practice. We may realize the full therapeutic potential of medicinal plants and make progress in the battle against viral infections for the good of humanity as we continue to elucidate the pharmacological mechanisms behind herbal antiviral activities.

Challenges and Strategies in Optimizing Herbal Formulations

Herbal medicine has been used for millennia to prevent and treat various ailments, but optimizing herbal formulations for safety, efficacy, and reproducibility presents unique challenges. Unlike conventional pharmaceuticals, herbal remedies often consist of complex mixtures of bioactive compounds with diverse chemical properties and pharmacological activities. Developing standardized herbal formulations that ensure consistent quality, potency, and therapeutic effects requires careful consideration of factors such as plant selection, extraction methods, formulation techniques, and quality control measures. This section will examine the methods and obstacles involved in optimizing herbal formulations, including formulation creation, quality control, standardization, and regulatory compliance, as well as ways to improve bioavailability. By addressing these challenges and adopting innovative strategies, researchers and manufacturers can improve the quality, safety, and efficacy of herbal medicines for the benefit of patients and consumers worldwide.

One of the primary challenges in optimizing herbal formulations is standardization, or ensuring consistency in the composition and potency of herbal products from batch to batch. Herbal medicines contain complex mixtures of bioactive compounds, which can vary widely in concentration depending on factors such as plant species, geographical origin, growing conditions, and harvesting practices. Standardization involves identifying and quantifying the active constituents or marker compounds in herbal extracts, establishing quality control specifications, and ensuring compliance with regulatory requirements. Gas chromatography-mass spectrometry (GC-MS) and also high-performance liquid chromatography (HPLC) are commonly used analytical techniques for phytochemical characterization and standardization of herbal extracts.

By standardizing herbal formulations based on marker compounds or bioactive constituents, manufacturers can ensure consistent quality and potency, enhance reproducibility, and improve the reliability of therapeutic outcomes.

Another challenge in optimizing herbal formulations is enhancing the bioavailability of bioactive compounds or the rate and also extent of absorption into the systemic circulation. Many plant compounds have low aqueous solubility, poor membrane permeability, and extensive first-pass metabolism, which can limit their bioavailability and therapeutic efficacy. Strategies for enhancing bioavailability include improving drug solubility, increasing membrane permeability, inhibiting metabolic enzymes, and promoting lymphatic absorption.

Formulation approaches such as nanotechnology, lipid-based delivery systems, microencapsulation, and complexation with cyclodextrins can improve the solubility, stability, and absorption of poorly soluble herbal compounds. Additionally, co-administration of absorption enhancers, enzyme inhibitors, or bioavailability enhancers can enhance the oral bioavailability of herbal extracts. By optimizing formulation strategies to improve bioavailability, researchers can maximize the therapeutic efficacy and clinical utility of herbal medicines.

Formulation development is a critical aspect of optimizing herbal formulations, involving the selection of excipients, dosage forms, and delivery systems that enhance drug stability, bioavailability, and patient acceptability. Herbal medicines can be formulated into various dosage forms, including tablets, capsules, powders, extracts, tinctures, teas, creams, ointments, and topical patches, depending on the route of administration, intended use, and patient preferences. Formulation techniques such as spray drying, freeze drying, lyophilization, hot melt extrusion, and supercritical fluid extraction are used to prepare herbal extracts with improved stability, solubility, and bioavailability. Additionally, innovative delivery systems such as liposomes, nanoparticles, microspheres, and transdermal patches can improve the targeted delivery of herbal compounds to specific tissues or organs, enhancing therapeutic outcomes and minimizing adverse effects. By optimizing formulation development, researchers can tailor herbal formulations to meet the diverse needs and preferences of patients, healthcare providers, and consumers.

From the selection of raw materials to the testing of the final product, quality control is crucial to guaranteeing the efficacy, safety, and consistency of herbal formulations throughout the production process. Herbal medicines are subject to contamination, adulteration, and variability in chemical composition, which can compromise product quality and safety. Quality control measures include identity testing, purity analysis, potency determination, microbial testing, and heavy metal screening of raw materials and finished products. Good manufacturing practices (GMP), quality management systems (QMS), and regulatory standards such as the United States Pharmacopeia (USP) and European Pharmacopoeia (Ph. Eur.) provide guidelines and requirements for quality control in herbal medicine manufacturing. Additionally, advanced analytical techniques such as nuclear magnetic resonance (NMR) spectroscopy, mass spectrometry (MS), and DNA barcoding can be used for authentication, traceability, and quality assurance of herbal products. By implementing robust quality control measures, manufacturers can ensure the safety, efficacy, and reliability of herbal formulations for consumers and patients.

Regulatory compliance is a significant challenge in optimizing herbal formulations, as herbal medicines are subject to varying regulations and standards in different countries and regions. Regulatory requirements for herbal products may include registration, licensing, labeling, safety assessment, efficacy evaluation, and post-market surveillance. In many jurisdictions, herbal medicines are regulated as dietary supplements, traditional medicines, or over-the-counter (OTC) products, with different requirements for product safety, efficacy, and quality control. Manufacturers must navigate complex regulatory frameworks and comply with relevant laws, regulations, and guidelines to ensure market access and product compliance. Collaboration with regulatory authorities, participation in industry associations, and adherence to international standards can facilitate compliance with regulatory requirements and promote consumer confidence in herbal products. Additionally, transparency, integrity, and accountability in product labeling, advertising, and marketing are essential for building trust and credibility with consumers, healthcare providers, and regulatory agencies.

Optimizing herbal formulations presents unique challenges and opportunities for researchers, manufacturers, healthcare providers, and regulatory authorities. Standardization, bioavailability enhancement, formulation development, quality control, and regulatory compliance are essential aspects of optimizing herbal medicines for safety, efficacy, and reproducibility. By addressing these challenges and adopting innovative strategies, stakeholders can improve the quality, accessibility, and acceptance of herbal medicines for patients and consumers worldwide. As interest in herbal medicine continues to grow, collaboration, communication, and cooperation among stakeholders will be essential for advancing the field, promoting evidence- based practice, and ensuring the responsible use of herbal remedies for the benefit of public health and well-being.

CHAPTER XI

Herbal Antivirals in Veterinary Medicine

Application of Herbal Therapeutics in Animal Health

Herbal medicine has been used for millennia to treat animal ailments; this technique is based on both empirical data and conventional wisdom. Humans have long noticed animals eating particular plants to cure illnesses or stay well, which has led to the discovery of certain botanicals' intrinsic therapeutic qualities. Herbal medicine is still a significant part of veterinary care today, providing supplementary or alternative treatments for a variety of ailments affecting cattle, wildlife, and companion animals.

Preventive care is one of the primary uses of herbal treatments in animal health. Herbal treatments are frequently utilized to strengthen the immune system, aid in digestion, improve nutritional condition, and shield animals against common health issues. Herbs that are known to stimulate the immune system, such as echinacea, astragalus, and garlic, can help the body respond more effectively to diseases and environmental stressors. Similarly, for companion animals as well as livestock, herbs like peppermint, chamomile, and ginger help promote digestive health and ease gastrointestinal disorders, including flatulence, diarrhea, and indigestion.

Caregivers can naturally promote their pets' general health and well-being by adding herbal supplements to their diets or daily routines. This lowers the risk of sickness and increases resilience to environmental obstacles.

In addition to traditional therapies, herbal remedies are frequently employed in veterinary medicine as supportive therapy to help animals with acute or chronic medical disorders manage their symptoms, reduce discomfort, and aid in their recovery. These treatments can enhance treatment outcomes, reduce side effects, and offer extra therapeutic benefits in addition to conventional medications. Herbs like arnica, calendula, and comfrey, for instance, are frequently applied topically to cattle and companion animals to relieve and treat wounds, cuts, and abrasions. Similar to this, animals who are agitated or nervous can benefit from the use of herbs like valerian, passionflower, and skullcap, which help to promote relaxation and lessen behavioral issues brought on by fear, separation anxiety, or noise sensitivity. Practitioners can offer comprehensive and customized treatment approaches that address the physical, emotional, and also mental well-being of animals, improving their overall quality of life and recovery by including herbal supportive therapies in veterinary care programs.

Herbal medicines are also being investigated more and more as complementary or alternative treatments for common veterinary ailments such as respiratory infections, gastrointestinal disorders, musculoskeletal diseases, and dermatological conditions. Herbal treatments can assist the body's natural healing processes and aid in an animal's recovery by offering symptomatic alleviation, antibacterial activity, anti-inflammatory effects, and tissue regeneration qualities. For example, anti-inflammatory and analgesic herbs such as devil's claw, Boswellia, and turmeric can aid older dogs or working animals with discomfort, stiffness, and inflammation related to arthritis, joint injuries, or musculoskeletal problems. Similar to this, expectorant, bronchodilator, and antibacterial qualities found in herbs like thyme, licorice, and mullein can benefit animals suffering from allergies or respiratory infections by reducing nasal congestion, sneezing, and coughing. Veterinarians may deliver efficient, individualized care that fosters healing, comfort, and well-being by customizing herbal remedies to each animal's unique requirements and situations.

However, there are drawbacks and things to think about when using herbal remedies for animal health. As botanicals contain bioactive components that might interact with pharmaceutical medications, physiological processes, and underlying health issues in animals, potentially causing harmful effects or drug interactions, one challenge is guaranteeing the safety and efficacy of herbal therapies. The safe and efficient use of herbal treatments in animals requires careful herb selection, dosage modifications, treatment response monitoring, and consultation with a licensed veterinarian. Additional factors to be taken into account to guarantee the quality, potency, and purity of herbal products for veterinary use include quality control, raw material procurement, manufacturing procedures, and product labeling. Veterinarians and other caregivers can optimize the advantages of herbal treatments while lowering risks and guaranteeing the health of the animals in their care by following best practices and evidence-based standards.

In summary, the use of herbal remedies in animal health presents exciting new possibilities for fostering wellness, treating illness, and improving animal welfare. Herbal medicines offer natural and holistic treatment choices that complement traditional veterinary medicine, ranging from supportive therapy and treatment of common animal illnesses to preventive care. By utilizing evidence-based practices and integrating herbal medicine into their practice, veterinarians can improve patient outcomes, expand treatment options, and promote the health and welfare of animals. The utilization of herbal medicine continues to rise in popularity, and in order to further the field and give our animal friends the best care possible, we must continue our research, teaching, and collaboration.

Comparative Aspects of Viral Diseases in Humans and Animals

Globally, viral illnesses cause a great deal of sickness, mortality, and economic losses, endangering both human and animal populations. Certain viruses can only infect people or animals; however, certain viruses can spread over species boundaries and cause zoonotic transmission, which can result in the formation of new diseases. Comprehending the similarities and differences between viral illnesses in people and animals is essential for deciphering the common etiology, locating zoonotic reservoirs, and putting into practice efficient measures for disease prevention, management, and surveillance.

The genesis of viral illnesses is an essential factor in both human and animal health. Numerous pathogens can cause viral disorders, including DNA viruses like herpesviruses and poxviruses, as well as RNA viruses like coronaviruses and influenza viruses. The degree of host specificity, tissue tropism, and transmission dynamics exhibited by these viruses affect their capacity to infect and disseminate within populations. Certain viruses are usually spread via direct contact, respiratory droplets, or bodily fluids; however, other viruses have a more comprehensive host range and can infect a variety of species, including people and animals. Animals are the original hosts of zoonotic viruses, which include rabies and avian influenza viruses. Humans can contract these viruses via direct contact with diseased animals, by consuming contaminated food or water, or by being exposed to polluted settings.

A number of variables, such as host population dynamics, environmental factors, and socioeconomic determinants, impact viral illness epidemiology in people and animals. Depending on their transmissibility, virulence, and geographic distribution, viruses can cause random outbreaks, localized epidemics, or worldwide pandemics. By changing host-vector interactions, natural environments, and social networks, factors like urbanization, deforestation, climate change, globalization, and human behavior can affect the origin and spread of viral illnesses. Zoonotic viruses can infect domestic animal populations after emerging from wildlife reservoirs. This can result in secondary transmission of the virus to humans via intermediary hosts or direct contact. The emergence of zoonotic diseases, including SARS-CoV, MERS-CoV, and SARS-CoV-2 (the agent responsible for COVID-19), emphasizes the need for cross-species surveillance and monitoring in order to identify and manage new infectious threats. These diseases also highlight the connection between human and animal health.

Viral components, host immune responses, and environmental factors interact intricately during the development of viral illnesses in people and animals, resulting in a variety of clinical presentations. Through particular receptor connections, viruses penetrate host cells, seize control of cellular processes to multiply and assemble new viral particles and elude host immune monitoring to establish infection. Numerous factors, including immunological conditions, host genetic susceptibility, virulence factors, and viral tropism, influence how a viral infection turns out. Certain viruses, like HIV and influenza A virus, frequently experience antigenic drift and shift, which can result in the creation of novel strains that are more transmissible, virulent, or resistant to vaccinations or antiviral medications. In order to cause spillover effects and persistent transmission in human populations, zoonotic viruses may go through reassortment processes or adaptive mutations in new host species.

Depending on the infecting virus, host species, age, immune system, and underlying medical conditions, the clinical signs of viral infections in humans and animals can differ significantly. Viral infections may trigger a wide variety of signs and symptoms, such as mild respiratory illness, fever, and fatigue, as well as severe pneumonia, encephalitis, hemorrhagic fever, and multiorgan failure. While some viruses, like herpesviruses and retroviruses, can create lifetime latent infections that occasionally reactivate to produce recurrent disease, others, like norovirus and rotavirus, predominantly target the gastrointestinal tract and cause diarrhea, vomiting, and dehydration. In contrast to their natural animal hosts, zoonotic viruses may present with distinct clinical symptoms in humans. These variations may be due to variations in viral tropism, immunological responses, and pathogenic processes.

Viral illnesses in humans and animals have severe consequences for public health, posing risks to social cohesion, food security, human health, and economic stability. Zoonotic viruses have the capacity to start pandemics, which could have a significant impact on socioeconomic advancement and the security of world health. The rise in zoonotic illnesses like COVID-19, Ebola, and Zika highlights the importance of early discovery, prompt action, and proactive surveillance in the face of new infectious dangers. In order to discover shared risk factors, prevent disease transmission and spread, and comprehend the complex dynamics of viral illnesses, One health approach that combines human, animal, and environmental health perspectives is crucial. In order to lessen the impact of viral infections and safeguard the health and well-being of humans as well as animals, collaboration between the healthcare industries for humans and animals is crucial. Proactive steps like immunization, biosecurity, and public health education are also essential.

Opportunities and Challenges in Integrating Herbal Medicine into Veterinary Practice

Veterinarians should think about the opportunities and obstacles associated with incorporating herbal medicine into their practice as they investigate complementary and alternative treatment alternatives for their patients. Herbal medicine has received recognition for its capacity to offer natural, holistic, and individualized care to animals. Its foundations are in empirical data and traditional knowledge. However, there are additional difficulties with safety, effectiveness, regulation, communication, and education when incorporating herbal medicine into veterinary care. Veterinarians who want to integrate herbal medicine into their clinical practice successfully must comprehend these opportunities and challenges.

The potential to increase treatment options and enhance patient outcomes is a significant advantage of incorporating herbal medicine into veterinary practice. Companion animals, livestock, and exotic species can all benefit from the alternative or supplemental therapies provided by herbal remedies for a variety of acute and chronic illnesses. Certain herbs, like echinacea, chamomile, and turmeric, are valuable supplements to treatment plans for ailments like dermatitis, arthritis, respiratory infections, and gastrointestinal disorders because of their anti-inflammatory, analgesic, antibacterial, and immunomodulatory qualities. Veterinarians can improve their patient's general health and well-being by tailoring treatment regimens to each patient's needs and preferences through the use of herbal medicine in their practices.

Furthermore, as pet owners and caregivers seek more natural and comprehensive methods of veterinary treatment, herbal medicine is in line with this trend. Given the possible hazards of side effects, drug combinations, and prolonged usage of synthetic treatments, a lot of pet owners are searching for substitutes for conventional prescription medications. For animals with sensitive constitutions or underlying medical disorders, herbal treatments provide mild, natural therapeutic options that frequently have fewer adverse effects. Furthermore, pet owners who value natural, eco-friendly, and cruelty-free goods for their pets may find herbal medicine intriguing as it aligns with the values of sustainability, environmental stewardship, and ethical animal care. Veterinarians can better serve their client's changing needs and preferences and increase their clients' happiness and loyalty by implementing herbal medicine into their practices.

In spite of the advantages, veterinarians need help with incorporating herbal medicine into their practice. These obstacles must be overcome to guarantee the safe, efficient, and moral application of herbal treatments. The absence of governmental control, evidence-based research, and defined recommendations for herbal products in veterinary care is a significant obstacle. Herbal products frequently lack standardized formulations, quality control procedures, and labeling standards, in contrast to pharmaceutical pharmaceuticals, which are subject to stringent testing, review, and regulation by governmental organizations like the U.S. Food and Drug Administration (FDA). Because of this, choosing the right herbs, figuring out the proper dosages, and guaranteeing product quality, purity, and potency can be complex tasks for veterinarians.

Veterinarians are forced to assess the safety and effectiveness of herbal medicines for their patients using their expertise, judgment, and experience in the absence of clear regulations and oversight.

Limited resources, training, and educational opportunities for veterinarians interested in integrating herbal medicine into their clinical practice present another obstacle to the integration of herbal medicine into veterinary practice. With a primary focus on conventional pharmacological therapy and surgical techniques, traditional veterinary school programs frequently offer limited exposure to herbal medicine. Consequently, many veterinarians need to be equipped with the information, abilities, and self-assurance needed to prescribe or deliver herbal medicines properly. Veterinarians' capacity to get specialized knowledge in veterinary herbal medicine is further hampered by the absence of approved training programs, continuing education opportunities, and certification alternatives in this area. The field of veterinary herbal medicine needs to be advanced, so veterinary schools and professional associations must create training programs, broaden their curriculum offerings, and encourage interdisciplinary collaboration between veterinarians, herbalists, botanists, and pharmacologist.

Additionally, in order to provide thorough and well-coordinated care for patients who are animals, veterinarians must collaborate and communicate with other medical professionals, such as herbalists, naturopaths, and holistic practitioners. Effective communication techniques are necessary to enable client talks regarding treatment alternatives, risks, benefits, and expectations when integrating herbal medicine into veterinary practice. Veterinarians need to tell their patients about the fundamentals of herbal therapy, possible drug interactions with prescription drugs, and the value of being open, truthful, and providing informed consent when making decisions. By building open, respectful, and mutually beneficial connections with their clients, veterinarians may help pet owners and caregivers make more informed decisions regarding the health and welfare of their dogs. This will increase the level of compliance, trust, and contentment with herbal treatment plans.

In conclusion, there are several opportunities to improve patient outcomes, increase the variety of therapies available, and meet the constantly changing requirements as well as preferences of caregivers and pet owners by integrating herbal medicine into veterinary care.

Herbal treatments offer alternative or supplemental therapies for a variety of acute and chronic ailments, giving animals personalized, natural, and holistic care. However, there are additional difficulties with safety, effectiveness, regulation, communication, and education when incorporating herbal medicine into veterinary care.

Veterinarians who want to overcome these obstacles need to keep up with the most recent findings, recommendations, and legislative changes pertaining to veterinary herbal medicine. To ensure the ethical and safe use of herbal medicines in veterinary practice, they must also work in conjunction with other healthcare professionals, educate clients about herbal medicine, and push for regulatory monitoring and standardized quality control methods. Veterinarians can improve the quality of life, health, and well-being of their animal patients by incorporating herbal medicine into comprehensive veterinary treatment. This can also lead to increased trust between clients and caregivers, contentment, and collaboration.

CHAPTER XII

Environmental and Sustainability Considerations

Impact of Herb Cultivation and Harvesting on Biodiversity

Ecological, social, and economic variables must all be carefully taken into account when analyzing the complex and varied question of how herb production and harvesting affect biodiversity. Herb farming has many advantages, such as more access to medicinal herbs, better financial prospects for farmers, and the preservation of wild populations; moreover, if conducted responsibly, there may be hazards to biodiversity. The impact of herb cultivation and harvesting on biodiversity is caused by a number of essential reasons, such as the introduction of invasive species, habitat degradation, overexploitation, genetic erosion, and disturbance of ecosystem dynamics.

The degradation of natural habitats and the conversion of natural ecosystems into agricultural land are two of the main issues with herb farming. Numerous therapeutic plants are indigenous to specific environments, including mountains, marshes, forests, and grasslands, where they are vital to the maintenance of ecosystem function and biodiversity. Removing native species, fragmenting landscapes, and losing essential habitats are all possible outcomes of clearing land for herb farming, which can lower biodiversity and diminish ecosystem services. The resilience and long-term sustainability of agroecosystems can also be jeopardized by the use of intense cultivation techniques, such as monoculture farming and mechanized agriculture, which can worsen habitat degradation and soil erosion.

Another significant danger to biodiversity is the overexploitation of wild plant populations, especially for species with limited distribution or high commercial value. Without proper management or supervision, many medicinal plants are taken from wild populations, which causes overharvesting, the loss of natural resources, and population decrease. Unsustainable harvesting methods can have catastrophic effects on biodiversity, including loss of genetic diversity, disturbance of ecological interactions, and increased susceptibility to environmental stressors. Examples of these methods include indiscriminate collection, habitat degradation, and the removal of entire plant populations. Conservation measures like the establishment of protected areas, the application of harvest quotas, and the promotion of sustainable harvesting practices are essential to minimizing the negative consequences of overexploitation on wild herb populations and preserving biodiversity.

Moreover, genetic erosion and biodiversity loss can be exacerbated by promoting the growth of commercially desirable or high-yielding varieties at the expense of genetic diversity in plant populations, herb cultivation, and harvesting. When choosing cultivars for cultivation, farmers in agricultural settings frequently give priority to qualities like productivity, uniformity, and disease resistance, which causes regionally adapted landraces and heirloom varieties to be displaced. Because of this, genetic diversity within farmed populations may gradually decrease, making plant populations less able to withstand changes in their environment as well as threats from pests and diseases. The long-term viability and resilience of agricultural systems depend heavily on efforts to conserve and enhance genetic variety in cultivated herb populations. Examples of these efforts include participatory breeding programs, on-farm conservation initiatives, and seed banking.

Herb farming and harvesting have direct effects on biodiversity, but they can also indirectly propagate invasive species and change the dynamics of ecosystems. Non-native herb species can upset native plant communities, displace native species in the competition for resources, and change the structure and function of habitats when they are introduced into new areas. It's possible for invasive herbs to escape cultivation and establish self-sustaining populations in their natural environments, which would degrade the habitat, eliminate native biodiversity, and interfere with ecosystem functions. Additionally, the distribution and abundance of native plant and animal species can be impacted by cultivation techniques, including fertilization, irrigation, and pesticide use, which can change the soil's composition, water availability, and nutrient cycling. Agroforestry, polyculture farming, and integrated pest control are examples of sustainable land management techniques that can lessen the ecological effects of herb agriculture and encourage the preservation of biodiversity.

In conclusion, a complex interaction of ecological, social, and economic factors affects how herb production and harvesting affect biodiversity. Herb farming has many advantages, such as better access to medicinal plants, financial gain for farmers, and preservation of wild populations; yet, if not conducted responsibly, there may be threats to biodiversity. Addressing these issues calls for an integrated strategy that incorporates ecological principles, conservation tactics, and stakeholder participation to maintain the long-term sustainability and resilience of herb-growing systems and maintain the long-term sustainability and resilience of herb-growing systems. We can lessen the adverse effects of herb cultivation on biodiversity and encourage the coexistence of agriculture and conservation by supporting sustainable land management techniques, preserving genetic diversity, controlling harvests, and encouraging cooperation between growers, researchers, legislators, and local communities.

Sustainable Practices in Herbal Medicine Production

In order to protect biodiversity, maintain the long-term viability and resilience of medicinal plant ecosystems, and advance the health and well-being of communities everywhere, sustainable practices in the production of herbal medicines are imperative. The cultivation, harvesting, processing, and distribution of herbal medicines are just a few of the many processes involved in their creation, all of which have an effect on the sustainability of the environment, society, and economy. Herbal medicine manufacturers can reduce environmental degradation, preserve natural resources, enhance biodiversity, and sustain local livelihoods by implementing sustainable practices across their whole supply chain. A number of important ideas and tactics, such as ethical sourcing practices, wildcrafting guidelines, agroecological farming techniques, quality control measures, fair trade initiatives, and community engagement programs, can guide sustainable herbal medicine production.

Because agroecological farming practices replicate natural ecosystems, improve soil fertility, conserve water, and use fewer chemicals, they are essential for increasing sustainability in the production of herbal medicines. Organic farming, permaculture, and agroforestry are examples of agroecological methods that place an emphasis on biodiversity, soil health, and ecological resilience while lowering the use of synthetic fertilizers, pesticides, and herbicides. Farmers may improve ecosystem services like pollination, pest control, and nutrient cycling while reducing environmental effects and boosting farm resilience to climate change by including medicinal plants in a variety of farming systems. By supporting local food systems, protecting traditional knowledge, and empowering small-scale farmers, agroecological farming also advances social justice and food sovereignty.

In order to ensure that medicinal plants are harvested sustainably from their natural habitats without affecting ecosystem integrity or biodiversity, wildcrafting rules are required. In order to reduce ecological consequences and encourage plant regeneration, wildcrafting, or the sustainable collection of wild plants depends on ideas like ethical stewardship, habitat conservation, and selective harvesting. Harvesting at the right time of year, avoiding overharvesting endangered species, leaving behind reproductive individuals, and honoring ecological and cultural sensitivity are only a few of the guidelines for wildcrafting. Furthermore, wildcrafters can collaborate with nearby communities, native populations, and land managers to create protected areas, set harvest limits, and carry out long-term management strategies for populations of medicinal plants. Herbal medicine makers can protect local people's rights and customs while guaranteeing the availability of wild plant resources for future generations by following wildcrafting standards.

By guaranteeing fair labor treatment, observance of human rights, and equitable benefit sharing along the supply chain, ethical sourcing procedures are essential to fostering sustainability and social responsibility in the herbal medicine sector. Transparency, accountability, traceability, and compliance with international labor norms, environmental laws, and indigenous rights are all part of ethical sourcing. In order to guarantee that manufacturers of herbal medicines follow moral principles and advance social justice, economic development, and cultural preservation in the areas where medicinal plants are sourced, fair trade initiatives, certification programs, and supply chain transparency methods can be helpful. Customers may aid in the empowerment of marginalized groups, sustainable development, and reduction of poverty in areas that produce herbal medicines by endorsing fair trade practices.

In order to minimize threats to the health and well-being of consumers while guaranteeing the safety, efficacy, and consistency of herbal medicine products, quality control methods are essential. Aspects of the manufacture of herbal medicines that fall within the purview of quality control include botanical identification, growth methods, harvesting strategies, processing processes, storage conditions, and labeling regulations. Furthermore, governmental supervision, quality assurance testing, and third-party certification programs can assist in confirming the efficacy, safety, and genuineness of herbal medicine items while shielding customers from contamination, adulteration, and mislabeling. Herbal medicine manufacturers can increase market competitiveness and advance public health by putting a high priority on quality control. This will help them gain consumers' confidence and establish credibility in their products.

In order to promote cooperation, empowerment, and shared stewardship of medicinal plant resources among stakeholders, such as farmers, wildcrafters, indigenous peoples, researchers, policymakers, and consumers, community engagement initiatives are crucial. In order to fulfill local needs, objectives, and aspirations, community-based methods for the development of herbal medicine involve participatory decision-making processes, knowledge exchange, capacity building, and resource sharing. Community gardens, farmer cooperatives, participatory research initiatives, and herbal medicine clinics can all be used as venues to support social inclusion, cultural diversity, and environmental sustainability in the manufacturing of herbal medicines. Stakeholders can improve collective action for sustainable development and the conservation of medicinal plant resources, foster social networks, and increase resilience by including local populations as active partners and participants in the manufacture of herbal medicines.

In conclusion, encouraging environmental stewardship, social fairness, economic development, and public health all depend on the use of sustainable production methods for herbal medicines. Herbal medicine producers can support biodiversity conservation, traditional knowledge preservation, community empowerment, and sustainable livelihoods by implementing agroecological farming techniques, wildcrafting guidelines, ethical sourcing practices, quality control measures, and community engagement initiatives. Working together, stakeholders such as farmers, wildcrafters, indigenous peoples, researchers, policymakers, and consumers can promote an inclusive, holistic approach to the development of herbal medicines that takes into account social, ecological, and economic factors. The herbal medicine sector may promote human and environmental well-being while guaranteeing the availability and accessibility of medicinal plants for future generations by adopting sustainability as a guiding concept.

Eco-friendly Approaches to Herbal Antiviral Research and Development

Research and development of herbal antivirals using environmentally safe methods is becoming more and more important as a means of tackling the double problems of preventing viral infections and reducing environmental damage. Conventional approaches for discovering antiviral drugs frequently depend on artificial substances produced through chemical synthesis, which can be resource-intensive, detrimental to the environment, and linked to negative consequences for ecosystems and human health. Eco-friendly methods, on the other hand, place more emphasis on organic, sustainable, and biodegradable solutions made from marine life, microbes, medicinal plants, and other renewable resources. Researchers can create safer, more effective, and environmentally sustainable antiviral medicines while reducing the ecological footprint of drug discovery and development procedures by utilizing the power of nature and implementing green chemistry concepts.

Using medicinal plants as a source of bioactive molecules with antiviral activity is one environmentally benign method of doing herbal antiviral research. Many traditional societies across the world have long used medicinal herbs to treat viral infections, modulate the immune system, and maintain overall health. Polyphenols, flavonoids, alkaloids, terpenoids, and essential oils are examples of plant-based antiviral chemicals that demonstrate a variety of pharmacological activities, such as antioxidant, immunomodulatory, antiviral, and anti-inflammatory properties. Researchers can find exciting candidates for additional study and development as antiviral medicines by screening plant extracts and bioactive chemicals against a panel of clinically relevant viruses. Furthermore, ethnobotanical research, phytochemical evaluations, and traditional knowledge systems can offer essential insights into the therapeutic potential, chemical makeup, and medicinal qualities of medicinal plants. These insights can direct drug discovery initiatives and support the conservation of biodiversity and cultural heritage.

The application of bioprospecting and bioprospecting to discover novel antiviral drugs from natural sources, such as microbes, marine organisms, and fungi, is another environmentally benign strategy for herbal antiviral research. Actinomycetes, bacteria, and fungi are examples of microorganisms that produce a wide range of bioactive substances with antiviral action, such as immunomodulators, antibiotics, and antifungals. Because of their distinct biochemical diversity and ability to adapt to harsh settings, marine creatures like algae, sponges, corals, and mollusks are also significant sources of bioactive chemicals with potential antiviral capabilities. Through the utilization of cutting-edge screening methods and the exploration of unexplored natural resources, scientists can find novel antiviral agents with distinct modes of action and therapeutic potential. In addition to supporting sustainable development and responsible environmental stewardship, bioprospecting initiatives can aid in biodiversity protection, ecosystem health preservation, and the sustainable use of natural resources.

The significance of green chemistry principles in drug discovery and development processes, such as the use of renewable feedstocks, solvent-free extraction techniques, biodegradable excipients, and environmentally friendly synthesis routes, is also emphasized by eco-friendly approaches to herbal antiviral research. Green chemistry seeks to minimize waste, cut down on energy use, and do away with dangerous compounds at every stage of the drug development process, from original discovery to production and disposal. Researchers can create antiviral medications with better safety profiles, fewer adverse effects on the environment, and more biocompatibility by using green chemistry concepts. This will result in more environmentally and socially responsible pharmaceutical goods. Furthermore, the pharmaceutical business may reduce its carbon footprint and hasten the transition to a circular economy that depends on closed-loop systems and renewable resources by utilizing green solvents, catalytic processes, and biobased components in its manufacturing.

Furthermore, in order to progress the field of natural product medication discovery and development, eco-friendly approaches to herbal antiviral research highlight the significance of interdisciplinary collaboration, knowledge exchange, and technology transfer between academia, industry, government, and civil society. The identification, characterization, and optimization of new antiviral compounds derived from natural sources can be facilitated by the interchange of expertise, resources, and best practices through collaborative research networks, consortia, and partnerships. Large datasets of chemical compounds, biological assays, and therapeutic targets can be accessed, analyzed, and shared by researchers with the help of open-access databases, bioinformatics tools, and high-throughput screening systems. These resources can accelerate the process of discovery. Eco-friendly methods for herbal antiviral research can accelerate the creation of new treatments for fighting viral infections while supporting social responsibility and environmental sustainability by encouraging a culture of cooperation, openness, and creativity.

To sum up, environmentally friendly methods of researching and developing herbal antivirals present encouraging prospects for reducing the worldwide incidence of viral infections, supporting sustainability, and avoiding adverse effects on the environment. Through the utilization of natural resources, the application of green chemistry principles, and the promotion of interdisciplinary cooperation, scientists can discover new antiviral compounds that are safer, more effective, and environmentally sustainable. Additionally, eco-friendly methods place a high priority on biodiversity conservation, traditional knowledge preservation, and fair benefit sharing. These strategies encourage responsible management of medicinal plant resources and the safeguarding of ecosystems and human health for future generations. Herbal antiviral research can help facilitate the shift to a more resilient and sustainable healthcare system founded on the values of social justice, ecological integrity, and economic prosperity by adopting eco-friendly methods and beliefs.

CONCLUSION

To fully realize the promise of herbal medicine in treating viral infections, "The Science of Herbal Antivirals: Emerging Trends in Natural Viral Defense Mechanisms" captures a voyage of discovery by fusing traditional knowledge with modern scientific investigation. During this investigation, we have uncovered the complex aspects of herbal antivirals by navigating the complex fields of virology, immunology, pharmacology, and ethnobotany.

Our research is motivated by a thorough understanding of the diverse array of compounds from plants that possess antiviral properties. The incredible endurance and adaptability of nature's pharmacy have been demonstrated by everything from current phytochemical investigations that have revealed novel bioactive compounds to ancient cures rooted in cultural heritage. Every chapter in this book is a tribute to the creative genius of herbalists, scientists, and healers from the past and present who have used plant power to combat viral dangers.

Upon contemplation of the knowledge acquired from these pages, it is clear there is still much work to do to fully comprehend herbal antivirals. The intricate interactions between plant chemicals and viral infections are still being uncovered by emerging research, opening up new possibilities for investigation and creativity. Similar difficulties and opportunities arise when integrating herbal medicine into conventional healthcare systems, necessitating a determined effort to close the gap between tradition and modernity.
Using herbal antivirals is more crucial than ever in light of international health emergencies like the COVID-19

pandemic. Herbal medicines are a valuable supplement to pharmacological interventions in managing disease, providing a comprehensive strategy that caters to the various needs of individuals and communities. We may increase our resistance to viral dangers by collaborating with herbalists, medical professionals, researchers, and policymakers to leverage the combined wisdom of traditional and scientific knowledge.

Let's keep our resolve to study herbal antivirals further as we get to the end of this voyage. By embracing new trends and harnessing the efficacy of natural remedies, we can pave the way for a future where everyone is healthier and more resilient.

Thank you for buying and reading/ listening to our book. If you found this book useful/ helpful please take a few minutes and leave a review on the platform where you purchased our book. Your feedback matters greatly to us.